EXERCISES IN
FETAL MONITORING

EXERCISES IN FETAL MONITORING

BARRY S. SCHIFRIN, M.D.

Director
Department of Maternal-Fetal Medicine
AMI Tarzana Regional Medical Center
Tarzana, California

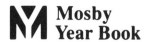

Mosby
Year Book

St. Louis   Baltimore   Boston   Chicago   London   Philadelphia   Sydney   Toronto

Mosby Year Book

Dedicated to Publishing Excellence

Sponsoring Editor: James D. Ryan
Associate Managing Editor, Manuscript Services: Deborah Thorp
Production Project Coordinator: Carol A. Reynolds
Proofroom Supervisor: Barbara M. Kelly

3 4 5 6 7 8 9 0 95 94 93 92

Library of Congress Cataloging-in-Publication Data
Schifrin, Barry S., 1938–
        Exercises in fetal monitoring/Barry S. Schifrin.
            p.   cm.
        Includes bibliographical references.
        ISBN (invalid) 0-8151-7565-6
        1. Fetal monitoring.   I. title.
        [DNLM: 1. Fetal Monitoring.   2. Heart Rate, Fetal.   WO 209 S333e]
RG628.S35   1990
618.3'2—dc20   91-12183
DNLM/DLC   CIP
for Library of Congress

Preface

For almost 20 years, electronic fetal monitoring (EFM) has been the mainstay of fetal surveillance before and during labor. Today the wide popularity of electronic fetal monitoring prevails despite different schemes of pattern interpretation and some controversy over its reproducibility and benefits. The controversy, however, cannot limit the obvious benefits of EFM and the increasing sophistication of interpretation of fetal heart rate (FHR) patterns. Confining the analysis of FHR patterns to a description of contraction-related events no longer suffices. We have come to understand that no single feature of the FHR pattern, such as type of deceleration or "dip area," suffices to encompass complex pathophysiologic responses, and that multifactorial analysis is necessary. Increasingly, this analysis focuses on the epochal fetal cardiac responses to various intrinsic and extrinsic provocations, including contractions. From such data we understand fetal patterns of behavior—even personality.

Electronic fetal monitoring has enhanced our understanding of fetal physiology and the breadth of cardiac responses to both asphyxial and nonasphyxial provocation. Electronic fetal monitoring predicts the absence of asphyxia with greater accuracy than any other known technique or combination of techniques. It has a lower false normal rate than fetal blood sampling (FBS) or auscultation. By this insight into the condition of the individual fetus, EFM has underscored the limitations of the clinical designations of "high-" and "low-risk pregnancy." Testing of the individual fetus is necessary to define its own risk status and may be viewed as the "well-fetus" examination.

It is widely claimed that EFM improves perinatal outcome, especially by reducing the risk of intrapartum stillbirth and low Apgar scores. The sudden, unexpected death of a fetus with a normal pattern has not been reported. Furthermore, outcome appears enhanced in both high- and low-risk patients. Anticipation, prevention, and timely intervention in fetal distress are the premise of monitoring; but the virtue of testing is to provide reassurance that fetal oxygen availability and neurological function appear to be sufficient in the presence of the stresses imposed by contractions (not labor), and that no intervention is necessary on behalf of the fetus. Electronic fetal monitoring patterns that contain a stable baseline rate, normal variability, and absent decelerations bespeak fetal well-being and cannot be counterfeited. Isolated movements and accelerations—fetal malaise—represent either an effect of medication, immaturity, or deterioration.

Electronic fetal monitoring has also facilitated considerably our ability to diagnose potential abnormalities. It provides insights into the mechanism of asphyxia and the likelihood with which such problems can be ameliorated with conservative management. In both the human and the experimental animal, we find an undeniable relationship between abnormal FHR patterns, hypoxia, low pH, and neonatal compromise. In addition, recently described patterns anticipate infants who will exhibit neonatal neurological abnormalities and subsequent handicap. Further, the information that EFM provides both before and during labor is simply unavailable from any other source.

Electronic fetal monitoring also has a number of limitations. It is far from being the perfect test system, and abnormal patterns cannot explain all untoward outcomes. Electronic fetal monitoring does not predict (nor does pH) neonatal distress resulting from trauma, sepsis, drugs, or congenital anomaly—factors that account for more than half of all cases of neonatal depression. Nor does EFM predict fetal distress very well as a number of apparently normal fetuses will demonstrate "abnormal FHR patterns." Electronic fetal monitoring does not reliably define growth retardation or congenital anomaly. In addition, the breadth of normal variation is considerable and not every deceleration is a step on the road to death. Ideally, the fetus would have a stable heart rate that decelerates only when threatened, and the greater the threat, the greater the deceleration. The complex and responsive fetus, however, does not lend itself to any simplistic, unidimensional approach. Electronic fetal monitoring patterns are not all quickly learned, and some patterns are not easily deciphered even after prolonged study.

Electronic fetal monitoring is further compromised by the absence of a uniform nomenclature. In addition, differences in technique (ultrasound or direct), scaling factors, and gestational age of the fetus have an impact on the interpretation of the tracing. These vagaries, along with the increasing use of EFM tracings in obstetrical malpractice cases and social forces demanding "natural birthing processes," have all conspired to increase the skepticism over the value of EFM.

The monitor cannot be used as a fancy stethoscope, nor can we compare the frequency of intervention for fetal distress as determined by EFM and auscultation. If the same criteria of distress used in auscultation are applied to EFM tracings, then the monitor is being misused, and the cesarean section rate will likely rise precipitously.

Considerable effort was involved in the reproduction of the tracings, and a brief explanation is necessary. The tracings, collected over the last 20 years, derive from my own patients as well as from those of other physicians and nurses who were kind enough to share with me what interested them. Still others derive from medicolegal cases. The original tracings were generated on a diverse group of fetal monitors, including some exotic and elaborate medical research equipment. Most of the FHR tracings were generated using scaling factors of 3 cm/min for the horizontal scale and 30 bpm for the vertical scale. Occasionally the 1 cm/min horizontal scale is used. For those in whom this is an infrequent and uncustomary scale, discipline will be necessary in assessing the tracing.

Irrespective of the source of the tracing, they were photographically separated from the original grid and reduced to about 45% of the original size. This tracing was then superimposed on a universal grid. The process is laborious, but I believe the results are worth the effort.

A simple experiment in optics will underscore my decision to use a colored grid. Without looking at the tracing, the reader should insert a finger between any two pages that contain tracings. Open the book for 1 second (no more than 2), look at the tracing, then immediately close the book. Most experienced readers will have some idea of the EFM pattern—reassuring or not. If the reader has entered into this experiment with the proper spirit, he or she will not have been able to determine the baseline heart rate. To illustrate this, repeat the exercise—this time looking at the tracing at leisure. Notice that the eyes are first drawn to the black line of the tracing and that the pastel grid is a blur. Because black and pastel are best seen in different parts of the eye, the eye must refocus to determine the heart rate from the grid.

This feature of optical physiology underscores the way tracings are read. As experience in reading tracings increases, the reader attempts to assimilate the whole pattern, paying less and less attention to the grid or to individual features of the tracing. Under normal circumstances, few experienced readers actually count the number or the amplitude of accelerations or decelerations. Focusing only on the most obvious features without a disciplined approach limits the amount of information that can be gleaned from the tracing.

An orderly approach to the analysis of the tracing has other virtues. It allows the interpreter to say something intelligent while stalling for time trying to figure out what the tracing means. In sequence the reader should assess (1) the baseline rate, (2) the stability of the baseline rate, (3) the baseline variability, (4) the presence of accelerations or decelerations in response to movement or contractions, (5) the impact of any deceleration on the baseline rate and variability and (6) the pattern of urerine contractions and fetal movement. By the time these descriptive features, which require no interpretation, are expounded, the diagnosis is usually obvious.

But to be able to read and interpret properly requires an understanding of fetal cardiac responses, an understanding of how the electronic fetal monitor operates, and a lexicon to be able to describe and communicate clearly.

This book is not designed as an introduction to EFM; numerous textbooks suffice for this purpose. Electronic fetal monitoring requires its own lexicon. The definitions and approach adopted here reflect a widely applied but by no means universally accepted standard. I encourage the reader to assess all aspects of the tracings and appraise not only the presence or absence of fetal hypoxia, but also estimate such features as gestational age, station, position, stage of labor, and pH from the clues available. Here, as under clinical conditions, the tracings are separate from the outcome results, and my own interpretations. While FHR tracings do not always permit accurate prediction of outcome, they always yield the opportunity for intelligent interpretation—and reasoned disagreement. As a generalization, the condition of the fetus and the difficulty of interpretation increase as the volume progresses.

Barry S. Schifrin

Acknowledgments

I wish to express my gratitude and indebtedness to those who have helped, encouraged, argued, and endured my frequent distractions. I make particular mention of nurses Marilyn Lapidus, Cyndi Afriat, Marilyn Steinberg, Kay Roll, Janie Jacobs, and Tina Hamilton. Drs. Wayne Cohen, Steve Myers, Richard Kates, Dan Clement, James Shields, and numerous other friends and colleagues too numerous to mention shared their ideas, their insights, and their skepticism. Finally, to my mother, wife, and children I express my love and gratitude for their sustaining love and forbearance.

Barry S. Schifrin, M.D.

Contents

Preface

ELECTRONIC FETAL MONITORING AND THE DIAGNOSIS OF FETAL DISTRESS

The term "fetal distress" is universally used to connote fetal hypoxia. No technique presently available, however, reliably predicts fetal hypoxia except in the terminally ill fetus. The value of newer techniques of electronic fetal monitoring (EFM) and fetal blood sampling (FBS) lies with the confident prediction of the nonasphyxiated fetus. Hypoxia is but one of several factors carrying the potential for fetal/neonatal compromise. Drugs, infection, trauma, and congenital anomaly may all contribute to low Apgar score, disordered neonatal adaptation, or subsequent disability or death without materially influencing FHR patterns or blood pH. For the most part, these nonasphyxial causes of low Apgar score cannot be determined reliably.

Fetal cardiac responses to hypoxia are varied. They depend not only on the rapidity of onset and the intensity of the asphyxial episode, but also on the frequency and intensity of uterine contractions. In the absence of significant uterine activity, the fetus will respond to slowly developing asphyxia with tachycardia—a response presumably mediated through discharge of sympathomimetic amines from the adrenal medulla. Under these conditions of minimal stress, tachycardia represents an early compensatory response to asphyxia. As the insult is prolonged, variability decreases. When compensation is no longer possible, the heart rate becomes unstable; it slows and death ensues. During labor, on the other hand, the earliest signs of distress are late or variable decelerations, which in turn are followed by rising heart rate and decreasing variability. If the asphyxial insult is acute and/or profound, the fetus will respond with bradycardia irrespective of contractions.

We have divided the clinical signs of fetal evaluation during labor into five categories: (1) reassuring, (2) suspicious, (3) threatening, (4) ominous, and (5) chronic. Each category consists of an evaluation of both baseline and periodic changes.

REASSURING PATTERNS

Early decelerations are not caused by hypoxia and do not appear to be associated with poor fetal outcome. Mild variable decelerations (often indistinguishable from early decelerations) appear totally innocuous, especially if associated with mild variable accelerations ("shoulders") before and after the deceleration. Uniform accelerations invariably signify a healthy reactive fetus. But most important, the presence of normal variability strongly suggests that there is no fetal indication for intervention.

SUSPICIOUS PATTERNS

Each of the baseline changes in the suspicious category may be associated with fetal hypoxia. But when such changes are not accompanied by decelerations, the mechanism is usually other than hypoxia. Clinically, maternal fever secondary to amnionitis is the most common discoverable etiology of fetal tachycardia. Here, the fetal and maternal rates rise in direct proportion to the fever. Frequently, a normal rate can be restored by prompt treatment of the underlying cause or by cooling the mother when the fever is excessive. Drugs, especially atropine and beta-sympathomimetics, may increase fetal heart rate. Fetal tachyarrhythmias may also be responsible for heart rate in excess of 180 bpm.

Baseline bradycardia, as opposed to a prolonged deceleration, is a late sign of fetal asphyxia. While babies who are about to die will invariably show bradycardia along with absent variability, the majority of babies with persistent heart rates below 120 bpm are not asphyxiated. Many babies with heart rates in the range of 90 to 120 bpm show no objective compromise. These babies usually demonstrate average baseline variability and absent decelerations. Baseline bradycardia in the range of 50 to 80 bpm may signal the presence of complete heart block. The latter can be diagnosed easily by fetal ECG analysis. Severely asphyxiated babies with bradycardia usually have sinus rhythm. Decreased variability may signify loss of fine autonomic (vagal) control of the heart rate from many causes. Decreased variability during labor may be seen with adequate oxygenation in premature fetuses, or when drugs are given to the mother during labor. All barbiturates, tranquilizers, and anesthetics, local or general, have the capacity for reducing variability. For these reasons we recommend that monitoring be commenced prior to the administration to the mother of any medication that has the potential for altering FHR patterns. Decreased variability in the absence of decelerations during labor is almost invariably related to an etiology other than asphyxia—usually medication. If an asphyxial insult is sustained by a baby whose heart rate variability is diminished by medications, decelerations will appear.

Suspicious patterns usually require no therapy. A search for the underlying cause should be made by stimulating the fetus. If hypoxia cannot reasonably be excluded, a fetal blood sample may be obtained. With a suspicious pattern, potentially compromising drugs or anesthetic techniques should be avoided until it is certain that factors other than hypoxia explains this pattern.

THREATENING PATTERNS

Threatening patterns represent unequivocal fetal response to impaired uterine blood flow (late decelerations) or impaired umbilical or intracranial blood flow (variable decelerations). While other mechanisms

4

have been proposed for these decelerations, their relationship to compromised blood flow is well established by clinical observation. Late decelerations associated with good variability appear during episodes of compromise in a baby with a previously normal pattern. We find this combination when the mother develops supine hypotension, with or without conduction anesthesia, and excessive uterine activity secondary to oxytocin. More important, these episodes are usually correctable with conservative measures. Improvement follows a predictable course. The baseline rate rises and variability diminishes as the amplitude of the deceleration diminishes then disappears. Subsequently, the baseline rate and variability return to normal.

The management of late decelerations includes (1) turning the patient on her side to eliminate supine hypotension and improve uterine blood flow, (2) administering oxygen by mask (5 L/min), (3) correcting of hypotension, if present, and (4) stopping oxytocin infusion.

In the majority of instances no obvious explanation for variable decelerations is found. However, the earlier they appear and the greater their frequency, the greater the likelihood of some obvious cord problem. Factors that increase the likelihood of variable decelerations include ruptured membranes, oligohydramnios, posterior position, vasa previa, nuchal cord, and short or prolapsed cord. As with late decelerations, we give little attention to the amplitude or, within reason, the duration of the deceleration, but rather judge the impact of the deceleration on the basis of the changes in baseline variability and rate associated with it. If baseline variability and rate remain stable, or only minimally affected, conservative maneuvers are implemented, and cesarean section is not performed.

Threatening patterns warrant measures directed at correcting the underlying disturbance in fetal or placental blood flow. In the majority of instances these patterns are correctable by eliminating oxytocin, turning the mother to the lateral position, and administering oxygen by face mask. Recovery can usually be anticipated. It is axiomatic that prevention is more important than therapy. Elimination of the supine position and judicious use of oxytocin infusion are appropriate safeguards in all patients. Administration of beta-sympathomimetics is gaining popularity as a temporizing measure in the treatment of fetal distress. Bicarbonate and glucose infusions are not of demonstrable value.

The response of variable decelerations to corrective measures is less predictable than the response of late decelerations. Often these patterns can be corrected or their severity reduced by manuevers designed to alter the geometric relationship between the fetus, cord, and uterine wall. Thus, altering the mother's positions between lateral, supine, Trendelenburg, and even knee-chest will frequently improve the pattern. But if we fail to relieve the pattern by such maneuvers, and intervention is considered, we attempt gentle elevation of the vertex. This maneuver,

however, should be undertaken only in the delivery room lest a prolapse of the cord be precipitated.

While variable decelerations are more common in the second stage of labor, the interpretation and therapy of the decelerations are the same in both first and second stages. Except when the head is crowning and delivery imminent, therapy should be governed by the conservative principles elaborated above, that is, by attempts at intrauterine resuscitation.

OMINOUS PATTERNS

Ominous patterns combine periodic features of the threatening category with the baseline patterns of the suspicious category. These patterns strongly suggest severe, acute distress of some duration. The mechanisms of these individual changes have already been discussed. Rebound accelerations ("overshoot") are uniform accelerations following variable decelerations of any amplitude and are accompanied by absent baseline variability. Baseline tachycardia is frequently associated with "overshoot" but preceding accelerations are usually absent. More than any other pattern, the combination of decreased variability and variable decelerations with "overshoot" strongly suggests autonomic imbalance. It may be seen following atropine administration or in premature or neurologically impaired fetuses and those severely asphyxiated.

An unstable rate with absent short-term variability that is occasionally "sinusoidal" is an added clue that fetal compensatory mechanisms have been exhausted. Such patterns have been reported in dying fetuses and those severely affected with Rh-isoimmunization. Cardiac denervation in the experimental animal produces a similar combination of unstable heart rate and absent short-term variability.

Sinusoidal patterns are not always ominous and are commonly seen after administration of narcotics to the mother.

Before fetal death only the ominous baseline changes may be present, and late or variable decelerations may be absent. Bradycardia is common at this time, but the rate may occasionally be found in the normal range. Heart rate changes in the terminally ill fetus are rarely dramatic. Cardiac arrest may occur, but unlike those episodes of asystole seen with variable decelerations, these are predictable, associated with sinus rhythm and are invariably fatal.

While the same conservative measures advocated for threatening patterns should be applied to the patient with ominous patterns, preparations should be made for expeditious delivery, as recovery is unlikely.

CHRONIC PATTERNS

A variant of the ominous pattern is one in which absent variability accompanies small variable decelerations with overshoot but late or severe decelerations are usually absent (no acute problem). The baseline rate is normal or elevated, and usually stable, the pH is usually in the normal range. Intervention is often employed, but is usually of little benefit.

INDICATION FOR INTERVENTION

While a number of fetal monitoring records demonstrate unequivocal fetal distress, intervention in the form of operative delivery is only rarely necessary. The indication for intervention on behalf of the fetus is "nonremediable" fetal distress. This philosophy represents an attempt to use the monitoring pattern to determine whether or not the maternal placental unit is capable of sustaining the fetus. With intact placental function and fetal blood flow, operative delivery does not appear warranted. The intact placenta is a faster, safer, and more efficient apparatus for resuscitating the fetus than is any man-made device. Under this concept no arbitrary time between onset of distress and optimal delivery is definable, nor can we safely state how much hypoxia is tolerable without compromise. If patterns of distress are not remediable, then intervention should be undertaken as quickly as is consistent with maternal and fetal safety.

TABLE 1.

Specificity Of FHR And FBS Indicators
Of Neonatal Depression

Cause of Depression	Specific FHR Pattern	Specific pH Pattern
Hypoxia	Late/variable decelerations	Acidosis
Congenital anomaly	Occasionally	None
Infection	Nonspecific	Nonspecific
Trauma	Nonspecific	Nonspecific
Drug	Nonspecific	Nonspecific

TABLE 2.

Fetal Heart Rate Responses To Asphyxia

	Uterine Contractions	
Asphyxial Insult	Present	Absent
Acute	Bradycardia	Bradycardia
Subacute/chronic	Late Decelerations	Tachycardia
	Variable Decelerations	

TABLE 3.

Classification Of Fetal Heart Rate Patterns

	Baseline Features	Periodic Features
Reassuring	Average variability	Absent decelerations
	Stable baseline rate	Early decelerations
		"Mild" variable decelerations
		Uniform accelerations
Suspicious	Tachycardia (>150 bpm)	Decelerations absent
	Bradycardia	
	Decreased variability	
Threatening	Average variability	Late decelerations
	Stable baseline rate	Variable decelerations
	Rising baseline rate	
Ominous	Absent variability	Late decelerations
	Unstable baseline rate	Variable decelerations with overshoot
	Bradycardia	
	Tachycardia	
Chronic	Absent variability	Variable decelerations with overshoot
	Tachycardia (>150)	

CAUSES OF FETAL ASPHYXIA

I. MATERNAL FACTORS

    A. Hypotension: hemorrhage, anesthesia, etc.
    B. Laryngospasm, aspiration.
    C. Anemia, high altitude, low O_2 mixtures.
    D. Functional pulmonary or cardiac disease.
    E. Fever (high), exercise (exhausting).
    F. Carbon monoxide, methemoglobinemia.

II. IMPAIRED UTERINE BLOOD FLOW

    A. Uterine contractions—uterine blood flow inversely proportional to uterine tone.
    B. Supine position—vena cava, aortic compression.
    C. Hypertension, diabetes, collagen diseases, etc.
    D. Vasopressors, local anesthetics.
    E. Ruptured membranes.

III. IMPAIRED UMBILICAL BLOOD FLOW

    A. Common during labor, especially second stage.
    B. Increased risk with oligohydramnios.
    C. Umbilical vessels sensitive to manipulation, cold, stretching, and local anesthetics.

D. Cord prolapse, hematoma, true knot.
E. Nuchal cord (probably need many loops).

IV. PLACENTAL FACTORS

A. Decreased area of exchange—abruptio, infarcts.
B. Increased thickness: erythroblastosis, lues, ? diabetes, ? inflammation, ? edema
C. Chronic placental insufficiency: may not be asphyxiated during labor.
D. ? Fever—increased consumption of oxygen.

V. FETAL FACTORS

A. Anemia:
  1. Abruptio, vasaprevia or placenta previa.
  2. Hemolysis, fetal-maternal hemorrhage.
B. Hydrops: acidotic during labor—not before.
C. Maternal hypotensive agents, diuretics.
D. Tachycardia, arrhythmia, anomaly.

LIMITATIONS OF CLASSICAL CRITERIA

I. CLINICAL AUSCULTATION OF THE FETAL HEART

A. Intermittent.
B. Confined to period between contractions.
C. Errors introduced:
  1. Technique.
  2. Listener bias.
  3. Variability.
  4. Decelerations.
  5. Accelerations.
D. Cannot assess:
  1. Variability.
  2. Type of deceleration.
  3. Recovery potential.
E. No value in predicting early fetal distress or subsequent outcome.

II. MECONIUM STAINING OF AMNIOTIC FLUID

A. Clinical correlations:
  1. Increased mortality and morbidity.
  2. "Normal" in breech presentation.
  3. Remains in amniotic fluid indefinitely.
  4. Many "normal" babies pass meconium.

B. Recent correlations:
  1. Related to fetal maturity, patent anus.
  2. Thickness a function of amniotic fluid volume.
  3. No increased incidence of ominous fetal heart rate (FHR) patterns or acidosis.
  4. Morbidity appears related to presence in neonatal respiratory tract (foreign body).
  5. Asphyxiated babies worse if meconium present.
  6. Need resuscitation personnel at delivery.
  7. Meconium aspiration may occur in utero—cannot prevent all meconium aspiration.
C. Intrapartum management:
  1. Presence requires FHR monitoring, and occasionally fetal blood sampling.
  2. Alone should not influence labor management.
  3. Demands personnel capable of neonatal resuscitation at delivery.

FETAL ACID-BASE BALANCE

I. DEFINITIONS

A. Acidemia—increased blood [H+] concentration.
B. Acidosis—increased tissue [H+] concentration.
C. Hypoxemia—decreased blood oxygen content.
D. Hypoxia—decreased tissue oxygen content.
E. Asphyxia—hypoxia and acidosis:
  1. Decreased pH, pO_2, HCO_3.
  2. Increased pCO_2, base deficit, lactate.

II. ENERGY, OXYGEN AND pH

A. Glucose is major energy source for fetus. With oxygen, glucose is metabolized to pCO_2 and H_2O, creating 38 moles of high-energy ATP for each mole of glucose.

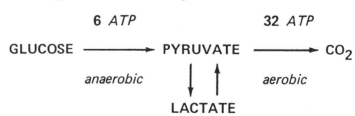

B. With sustained interruption of oxygen, glucose is not efficiently metabolized.
  1. Energy crisis—cost of energy increases; requires 6 moles glucose for same ATP.

2. Build up of lactate, other (fixed) acids; fall in pH—*metabolic acidosis.*
3. Acidosis poisons enzyme systems.
4. Slowly correctable.
C. With brief interruption of oxygen (e.g., cord compression):
1. Acute fall in pH from build up of CO_2—*respiratory acidosis.*
2. No increase in lactate or fall in HCO_3.
3. Analogous to breath holding in adults.
4. Rapidly correctable.

III. ACID-BASE PARAMETERS

A. pH
1. The negative logarithm of the hydrogen ion [H+] concentration.
2. A measure of oxygen availability to the fetus.

$$\propto \frac{METABOLIC\ COMPONENT}{RESPIRATORY\ COMPONENT}\quad \frac{HCO_3^{-}\ (BD)}{pCO_2}$$

B. pCO_2—respiratory component:
1. Partial pressure of CO_2 in blood.
2. Separate respiratory, metabolic acidosis:
   Increased pCO_2—respiratory acidosis.
   Normal pCO_2—metabolic acidosis.
C. Base deficit (BD)—metabolic component:
1. Similar to buffer base (BB).
2. A measure of bicarbonate deficit.
D. pO_2
1. Partial pressure of oxygen in blood.
2. Not reliable estimate of oxygen availability—hemoglobin saturation and blood flow better.
3. Low values in normal babies and vice versa.
E. Normal values:
1. pH: 7.25–7.40.
2. pCO_2: 35–45 mm Hg.
3. Base deficit: 4–7 mEq/L.
4. pO_2: 20–30 mm Hg.
F. Action values (Saling):
1. Normal: >7.25.
2. Pre-acidotic: 7.20–7.24.
3. Acidotic: <7.20.

IV. CAUSES OF FETAL ACIDEMIA

A. Fetal asphyxia.
B. Maternal acidemia.
C. Drugs, especially ritodrine and terbutaline.

V. CORRELATION WITH HEART RATE PATTERNS

A. Poor correlation between pH and baseline rate.
B. Fetal acidosis with ominous pattern.
C. Confirm mechanisms of decelerations.
D. Absent acidosis with reassuring patterns.

FETAL BLOOD SAMPLING

A. Technique
1. Cervix dilated 2 to 3 cm; −1 station.
2. Position—lithotomy or lateral Sims.
3. Sterile setup—introduce endoscope.
4. Create seal to prevent contamination—fundal pressure may help.
5. Dry scalp with swab; apply silicone.
6. Puncture scalp with guarded blade (2 mm) at right angles to scalp; 3 punctures maximum.
7. Collect blood in heparinized tube—suction if necessary.
8. Seal tube, mix blood, chill and analyze.
9. Visualize site during next contraction.
B. Clinically
1. Need FHR monitoring to determine who requires sampling. Attempt correction first.
2. Most high-risk fetuses have normal pH in early labor; don't need baseline pH.
3. Normally, no fall in pH during first stage of labor. Moderate drop during second stage—preventable with lateral position.
4. Significant asphyxia always lowers the pH.
5. *Metabolic acidosis*—develops slowly; requires about two to four times as long to recover—a "good memory" system.
6. *Respiratory acidosis*—develops and recovers quickly; a "poor memory" system.
7. Need serial samples to determine recoverability.
8. Samples best obtained between contractions.
9. Samples easiest to obtain during contractions.
C. Indications
1. Unclassified pattern or uncertain diagnosis.
2. Absent variability without decelerations.
3. Late decelerations with good variability.

4. Not much help with variable decelerations. If you do, attempt sample before next contraction.
5. Unnecessary with benign or ominous patterns.
6. Meconium.
D. False negative—normal pH/poor outcome.
1. Less than 50% of babies depressed at birth can be accounted for on basis of low pH.
2. Long interval between sample and delivery.
3. Technical problem, sampling error.
E. False positive—low pH/normal outcome.
1. Sample taken during variable deceleration.
2. Respiratory acidosis or maternal acidemia.
3. Long interval between sample and delivery.
4. Technical problem, sampling error.
F. Complications
1. Hemorrhage—determine bleeding source after sampling. Control with clip if necessary.
2. Hematoma, infection of scalp.
3. Precipitate or correct variable decelerations.
4. Precipitate supine hypotension, late decelerations.
G. Pitfalls
1. Position awkward for patient and physician.
2. Patient immobile, lithotomy position unphysiologic.
3. Need serial determinations.
4. Source of blood, speed of flow, etc.
5. Easiest time to collect blood is during a contraction; this is also the time when decelerations develop.
6. *Baseline* pH is more important than *periodic* pH.
7. Generally determine only pH; does not separate respiratory from metabolic acidosis—need pCO_2.
8. Inability to obtain sample (about 10% of the time).
a. Peripheral vasoconstriction—sick fetus.
b. Scalp edema, "hairy scalp."
9. Misinterpretation of results.
H. Practicality
1. Indispensable technique—research.
2. Useful technique:
a. Large service, experienced personnel.
b. Technical support.
3. Limited value:
a. Small service, inexperienced personnel.
b. No technical support.

BASELINE HEART RATE

DEFINITIONS
A. Normal range: 110–150 bpm
B. Tachycardia: >150 bpm
C. Bradycardia: <110 bpm
D. Baseline—refers to events between contractions.

TACHYCARDIA
A. Etiology
1. Asphyxia
2. Idiopathic
3. Maternal fever
4. Fetal infection
5. Prematurity
6. Drugs, e.g., atropine, isoxsuprine
7. Arrhythmia
8. Maternal anxiety
9. Maternal thyrotoxicosis
B. Clinically
1. Bimodal distribution of outcome in babies with tachycardia.
a. Absent decelerations, generally good outcome.
b. With late/variable decelerations, generally poor outcome.
2. Fetal tachycardia sometimes precedes maternal fever; degree of tachycardia proportional to fever.
3. Tachycardia not good indicator of severity of fetal infection.
C. Management of tachycardia
1. Rule out maternal cause (fever) or drug effect.
2. Rule out fetal arrhythmia.
3. If associated with late or variable decelerations—(see Treatment of Fetal Distress near the end of this outline).
4. Intervention probably not warranted for tachycardia per se (some disagreement on this point).
5. Notify pediatrician. Tachycardia may cause heart failure in newborn.

BRADYCARDIA
A. Etiology
1. Asphyxia—late
2. Arrhythmia
3. Drug effect
4. Hypothermia

B. Clinically
   1. Many normal babies with heart rate in range from 90 to 110 bpm.
      a. Normal variability.
      b. Absent decelerations.
   2. Must consider congenital heart block in differential diagnosis; rate usually 50 to 70 bpm, absent variability.
   3. Make certain that bradycardia is fetal, not maternal.
   4. A very late sign of fetal asphyxia:
      a. Flat heart rate.
      b. Late decelerations may be absent.
C. Management
   1. Rule out fetal death.
   2. Obtain fetal ECG—rule out congenital heart block.
   3. With good variability and absent decelerations—observe.
   4. If associated with decreased variability and/or decelerations—ominous

BASELINE VARIABILITY

LONG-TERM VARIABILITY

A. Definition—fluctuations in heart rate measured over many seconds.
B. Characteristics
   1. Amplitude
      a. Increased: >15 bpm
      b. Average: 5 to 15 bpm
      c. Decreased: <5 bpm
      d. Absent: <2 bpm
   2. Frequency
      a. 2 to 6 cycles per minute.
      b. Occasionally sinusoidal.

SHORT-TERM VARIABILITY

A. Definition—interval (or rate) differences between successive heartbeats.
B. Characteristics—not well defined.
   1. Amplitude range—0 to 40 bpm.
   2. Frequency—probably in range of 20 to 60 cycles per minute average.
   3. Average interval difference—about 5 msec.
   4. Changes are unpredictable.

UNDERLYING MECHANISMS

A. Long-term variability reflects interaction between influences that increase rate (sympathetic) and influences that decrease rate (parasympathetic).
B. Short-term variability reflects vagal efferent traffic only.
C. Presence of variability suggests adequate CNS control over FHR.

CLINICALLY

A. "Normal variability" refers to "normal short-term variability." "Poor variability" refers to "poor short-term variability."
B. Use presence of short term variability as indicator of fetal reserve. Look to deceleration waveform for mechanism of insult.
C. Majority of babies with good short-term variability do well regardless of decelerations present.
D. Majority of babies with diminished variability have good outcome if there are no associated decelerations.
E. Virtually all babies with significant asphyxia and all babies who are about to die will have decreased/absent variability.
F. Asphyxia is not the most common cause of decreased variability.

DECREASED VARIABILITY—Etiology

A. Asphyxia.
B. Drugs.
   1. Atropine—scopolamine.
   2. Tranquilizers—diazepam.
   3. Narcotics.
   4. Barbiturates.
   5. Local anesthetics.
C. Prematurity.
D. Tachycardia.
E. Physiologic "sleep."
F. Anesthesia.
G. Cardiac and CNS anomalies.
H. Arrhythmias—especially nodal rhythm.

INCREASED VARIABILITY (SALTATORY PATTERN)

A. Usually found following moderate-severe variable decelerations—probably reflects period of cardiovascular readjustment.
B. Unrelated to variable deceleration.
   1. Coalescence of accelerations with fetal movement.
   2. Highly reactive autonomic nervous system.
C. No therapy recommended—but anticipate variable decelerations.

PITFALLS

A. In the majority of instances, long- and short-term variability increase and decrease together. In some instances, may have one without the other.

B. When speaking of good and poor variability, we are referring to short-term variability only.

C. The presence or absence of long-term variability should not modify the interpretation.

D. These discussions apply only to baseline variability and not to the changes in variability during a deceleration or contraction.

E. Technical—all that wiggles is not variability (see technical section).

SINUSOIDAL HEART RATE PATTERN

A. Sine wave characteristics.
   1. Period—time required for one cycle.
   2. Frequency—number of cycles per unit time, e.g., cycles per second = hertz (Hz).
   3. Period = 1/frequency.
   4. Amplitude—maximum height of sine wave.

B. Relationship to FHR patterns.
   1. Few, if any, FHR patterns are exactly like above; hence the designation sinusoidal.
   2. Thus far, little attention paid to above characteristics.
   3. Usual features of patterns reported thus far:
      a. Amplitude—5 to 15 bpm (some greater).
      b. Frequency—2 to 5 cycles per minute (cpm).
      c. These characteristics same as normals.

C. Clinical classification of sinusoidal patterns.
   1. Ominous pattern—usually intermittent.
      a. Rh isoimmunization.
      b. Other high risk—e.g., toxemia.
      c. Terminal pattern.
   2. Benign pattern—reactivity elsewhere.
      a. Normal outcome.
      b. No identifiable cause.
   3. Compensatory—following severe variable decelerations.
   4. Cardiac anomaly.
   5. Sepsis.
   6. Other.

D. Intervention probably not indicated solely on basis of sinusoidal pattern.

EARLY DECELERATIONS

A. Characteristics.
   1. Shape—uniform.
   2. Onset—coincident with onset of contraction.
   3. Lag time—less than 20 seconds.
   4. Duration—proportional to duration of contraction.
   5. Amplitude—proportional to amplitude of contraction.
   6. Repetitive.

B. Proposed mechanism.
   Head (fontanelle) compression
   > Increased intracranial pressure
      > Increased peripheral resistance
         > Increased blood pressure
            > Reflex (vagal) deceleration

C. Clinically.
   1. Common during second stage and in primigravidas.
   2. Exaggerated with forceps application.
   3. Benign pattern.

D. Observations.
   1. Unaffected by position change or oxygen administration.
   2. Abolished by atropine.
   3. Not associated with alterations in baseline heart rate or acid-base balance.

LATE DECELERATIONS

A. Characteristics.
   1. Shape—uniform.
   2. Onset—late in contraction cycle.
   3. Lag time—greater than 20 seconds.
   4. Duration—proportional to duration of contraction.
   5. Amplitude—proportional to amplitude of contraction.
   6. Repetitive.

B. Proposed mechanism.
   Diminution in uterine blood flow with contraction
   > Critical reduction of pO_2 during peak of contraction
      > Reflex slowing (vagal) of heart rate (central)
         > Hypoxemia of myocardium (local)

C. Clinically.
   1. Associated with obstetrical/anesthetic procedures.
      a. Supine hypotension.
      b. Epidural/spinal anesthesia.
      c. Excessive uterine activity.
   2. Placental insufficiency.
      a. Intrauterine growth retardation.

b. Hypertensive disorders of pregnancy.

c. Other causes.

D. Observations.

1. Effect of position change—may improve pattern if it is related to supine hypotension.

2. Effect of atropine

a. Atropine may increase baseline rate and diminish variability and as a result, alter the amplitude of the decelerations.

b. Atropine does *not* eliminate the deceleration.

3. Effect of oxygen.

a. May diminish or abolish deceleration pattern.

b. It is uncertain whether administration of oxygen improves fetal acid-base abnormalities.

c. Wean patient off of oxygen before resuming management.

4. Baseline changes.

a. Diminished variability.

b. Tachycardia—common, but not inevitable, feature.

5. Acid-base balance changes.

a. Little change initially—in previously normal fetus, late decelerations precede changes in acid-base balance.

b. If deceleration present for 20 minutes or more, will usually find acidosis.

c. Acidosis proportional to severity and duration of decelerations.

d. *But,* for given amplitude and frequency of late decelerations, acidosis less with good variability than with poor variability.

VARIABLE DECELERATIONS

A. Characteristics.

1. Shape—variable

2. Onset—variable

3. Lag time—variable

4. Amplitude—variable; usually unrelated to amplitude and duration of contraction

5. Need not be repetitive

6. Frequently preceded or followed by brief variable accelerations (shoulders)

B. Proposed mechanism.

Umbilical cord occlusion (spasm)

> Increased peripheral resistance

> Increased blood pressure

> Stimulation of baroreceptors/chemoreceptors

> Reflex (vagal) deceleration—(initial)

> Hypoxia

> Bradycardia—(late)

C. Clinically.

1. Most common pattern observed (about 40% of all monitored babies).

2. High incidence in fetuses with:

a. Nuchal cord.

b. Short or prolapsed cord.

3. In majority of instances, however, no obvious explanation for variable deceleration patterns is found.

4. More common if membranes are ruptured than if intact.

5. Deceleration corrected or precipitated by manipulations, e.g., vaginal examination, alteration of maternal position, or scalp sampling.

D. Observations.

1. Effects of position change.

a. May correct pattern.

b. May precipitate pattern.

2. Effects of atropine.

a. Delays onset of deceleration.

b. May obliterate brief deceleration.

c. Diminishes abruptness of slope of deceleration.

d. Accentuates rebound accelerations.

e. Increases baseline rate—diminishes variability.

3. Effect of oxygen—*none.*

4. Arrhythmias.

a. Because of profound vagal stimulus from cord compression, there is suppression of S-A node. As a result, may find a number of changes in cardiac rhythm.

b. Nodal rhythm.

1. Probably most common arrhythmia in fetus.

2. Variability invariably absent during nodal rhythm.

3. Document with ECG—absent P waves.

c. May have transient cardiac arrest (heart block); usually seen at the base of the variable deceleration.

d. Ventricular escape beats—premature ventricular beats

e. *Sudden death during variable deceleration virtually unheard of—not indication for intervention.*

5. With increasing severity of pattern:

a. With resilient fetus:

1. Moderate to severe variable decelerations may be accompanied by an erratic rebound acceleration and average to increased baseline variability.

b. In deteriorating fetus:
   1. Variable accelerations (shoulders) disappear.
   2. Rising heart rate and diminishing variability.
   3. "Peaked" shoulders follow deceleration.
   4. Descent becomes less abrupt.
   5. Recurrent rebound accelerations (overshoot)—ominous feature.
c. Judge severity of deceleration not by duration or amplitude, but by impact on baseline rate and variability.
6. Acid-base balance changes:
   a. pH may decrease dramatically during deceleration.
   b. This is primarily respiratory acidosis due to acute buildup of carbon dioxide.
   c. As soon as circulation re-established, carbon dioxide cleared and pH returns to normal.
   d. Acidosis is proportional to effect on baseline rate and variability.
   e. Need to obtain pH sample between decelerations to determine impact on fetus.

PROLONGED DECELERATIONS

A. Characteristics.
   1. Onset—abrupt.
   2. Amplitude—at least 30 bpm.
   3. Duration—at least 2 minutes.
   4. Not homogeneous group of patterns—vary considerably in:
      a. Rapidity of onset.
      b. Relationship to uterine contractions.
      c. Rapidity of recovery.
      d. Patterns during recovery.
      e. Duration and amplitude.
   5. Must distinguish from baseline bradycardia.
B. Proposed mechanism.
   1. Uncertain.
   2. Most probably reflex (vagal) in origin—at least initial part of deceleration.
   3. Potential for developing hypoxia if prolonged.
   4. Predisposing causes—not always obvious.
      a. Uterine hypertonus.
      b. Manipulation.
         1. Vaginal examination.
         2. Scalp sampling.
         3. Position change.
      c. Drugs—especially with frequent uterine contractions.

C. Clinically.
   1. Prolonged decelerations occur most commonly during the second stage—but may appear at any time.
   2. Majority of babies with these decelerations will be delivered in good condition.
   3. Anticipate recovery if preceded by normal variability or variability present within deceleration.
   4. Anticipate intervention if previous pattern abnormal, or deceleration persists without variability for over 3 minutes.
D. Acid-base balance changes.
   1. If deceleration prolonged, almost always get acidosis.
   2. Recovery from acidosis trails behind rate recovery.
   3. Only sequential blood sampling will be of clinical benefit.
E. Management.
   1. Interpretation and therapy of these decelerations should be the same regardless of stage of labor.
   2. Delivery not necessarily the best course of management, despite the fact that baby is "deliverable."

COMBINED DECELERATIONS

A. Characteristics.
   1. Combination of two deceleration patterns (e.g., early/late; early/variable; variable/late)
B. Proposed mechanism—See individual deceleration patterns.
C. Clinically.
   1. Unusual patterns.
   2. Treat according to most ominous pattern.
D. Pitfalls.
   1. Slow recovery from variable deceleration—not the same as combined variable/late deceleration.
   2. Must be able to demonstrate substantially *both* waveforms.

SPORADIC/UNCLASSIFIED DECELERATIONS

A. Sporadic.
   1. Decelerations unrelated to contraction.
   2. Majority have appearance of variable decelerations.
   3. Usually short-lived and appear with otherwise reassuring FHR patterns.
   4. Appear to have little clinical significance.
B. Unclassified decelerations.
   1. Decelerations whose waveform characteristics preclude classification into early or late decelerations.
   2. Examples.
      a. Early onset, late return, uniform deceleration.
      b. Late deceleration preceded by acceleration.

c. Isolated late or early deceleration. Although waveform is typical of late deceleration, it does not repeat with contractions of similar amplitude. Early and late decelerations are proportional to amplitude and duration of contractions.

   3. Management.
      a. With good variability—therapy unnecessary.
      b. With poor variability—scalp sample if possible.
   4. Consider congenital anomaly.

ACCELERATIONS

A. Spontaneous accelerations.
   1. Uniform, symmetrical accelerations unassociated with contractions or periodic decelerations.
   2. Seen with fetal movement or stimulation.
      a. Represents integrative response of fetal CNS.
      b. Basis of reactive NST.
   3. Apparently benign response.
B. Uniform accelerations.
   1. Uniform, symmetrical acceleration.
      a. Coincident with uterine contractions.
      b. Reflects shape of contraction.
   2. Occurrence.
      a. Early in labor—before membranes ruptured.
      b. Following atropine administration.
      c. Common in nonvertex presentations.
   3. Apparently benign response.
C. Variable accelerations.
   1. Variably shaped accelerations that do not reflect shape of uterine contraction.
      a. "Shoulders" on variable decelerations.
      b. As feature of "increased variability" with contractions.
      c. Usually associated with good baseline variability.
   2. Apparently benign response.
D. Rebound accelerations (overshoot).
   1. Uniform accelerations following variable decelerations.
   2. Characteristics.
      a. Smooth baseline.
      b. Follows variable deceleration regardless of amplitude.
      c. Usual duration—longer than 12 seconds.
      d. May also be seen:
         1. Following administration of atropine.
         2. Immature fetus.
      e. Do not confuse with exaggerated variable acceleration following moderate-severe variable deceleration.
   3. Ominous commentary on variable deceleration.

TABLE 4.

Accelerations Associated With Variable Decelerations

	"Shoulders"	"Overshoot"
Occurrence	Precedes and/or follows variable decelerations; may vary from contraction to contraction	Follows variable decelerations; consistent; recurrent
Duration	Usually <12 seconds	>12 seconds
Baseline variability	Usually average; sometimes increased	Absent
Fetal condition	Usually good	1. Severely asphyxiated 2. Prematurity or immaturity 3. Following atropine administration
Proposed mechanism	1. Minor degree of slowly developing umbilical cord compression (venous) 2. Interaction of sympathetic and parasympathetic systems	Impairment of vagally mediated control mechanism

EFFECTS OF DRUGS ON FETAL HEART RATE

A. General principles—must consider.
   1. Direct effect on fetus:
      a. Most drugs cross placenta.
      b. Including: narcotics, anesthetics, etc.
      c. Exceptions: heparin, succinylcholine, et al.
   2. Maternal hemodynamics:
      a. Blood pressure (BP).
      b. Total peripheral resistance (TPR).
      c. Cardiac output (CO).
      d. Affected by maternal position.
      e. Effects may be indirect (e.g., anxiety).
   3. Uterine contractility, blood flow (UBF).
B. Tranquilizers/sedatives, etc.
   1. Decreased baseline variability—vagolytic effect (e.g., diazepam, meperidine, phenobarbital, etc.).
   2. If fetus hypoxic will develop decelerations.
C. Autonomic agents.
   1. Atropine:
      a. Decreases variability.
      b. Increases heart rate—rarely over 160 bpm.

c. Induces accelerations during contractions.

d. Obliterates early decelerations.

e. Modifies variable decelerations: smooth decelerations with "overshoot."

f. Little effect on late decelerations.

2. Beta-adrenergic blockers (propranolol, etc.):
   a. Decrease rate (proportional to baseline).
   b. Decrease variability.
   c. Decelerations with UC (vertex).

3. Beta-adrenergic stimulants (terbutaline, ritodrine):
   a. Decrease variability.
   b. Increase rate.
   c. Beat-to-beat arrhythmia.
   d. Similar changes in mother.

4. Ephedrine:
   a. May increase baseline rate.
   b. Increase variability (saltatory pattern).
   c. Corrects hypotension—ameliorates distress.

D. Oxytocin.

1. With careful control, uterine activity similar to spontaneous labor. Differences:
   a. Faster labors.
   b. Regular contraction interval and amplitude.
   c. Coupling of contractions.

2. Physiologic range—1 to 16 mU/min:
   a. Short half-life of drug.
   b. Some uteri exquisitely sensitive.
   c. Use constant-infusion pump.
   d. Start at low rate: 0.5 to 1.0 mU/min.
   e. Don't increase infusion rate more often than every 30 to 60 minutes.

3. Excessive stimulation:
   a. Tachysystole/hypertonus/tetany.
   b. Fetus determines excessive activity.

4. Oxytocin does not cross placenta. Effect on fetus secondary to effect on uterine blood flow (UBF).

E. Local anesthetics.

1. Ester-linkage (e.g., procaine): Don't cross placenta.
2. Amide linkage (e.g., lidocaine)—cross placenta.
3. Drugs appear in fetus—poorly metabolized.
4. Direct cardiac toxicity with massive dosage.
5. Effects on uterine contractions:
   a. Increased then decreased contractility.
   b. Occasionally hypertonus and tachysystole.
   c. Oxytocin augments hypertonus.

d. Oxytocin does not prevent decrease in uterine contractility.

6. Post PCB bradycardia may represent:
   a. Effect on fetal CNS.
   b. Uterine hypertonus, tachysystole.
   c. Direct effect on myocardium—unlikely.
   d. Beat-to-beat arrhythmia.
   e. Effect on uterine/umbilical vessels.
   f. Manipulation.
   g. Use of epinephrine.

7. Maternal convulsions after I.V. injection.

8. Maternal hypotension after epidural.

9. Drugs appear in maternal and fetal circulation irrespective of injection site.

FETAL DISTRESS

A. Phases of asphyxial insult during labor.

1. Asphyxial insult—must have:
   a. Late or variable decelerations associated with rise in baseline, decrease in variability.
   b. Prolonged decelerations, sudden bradycardia.

2. Recovery:
   a. Period between end of insult and return to stable baseline rate and variability.
   b. May recover with or without residual.
   c. Duration: 2 to 4 times duration of insult.

3. Recovery without residual (sequence may vary):
   a. Decelerations diminish.
   b. Baseline rises, variability decreases.
   c. Decelerations disappear.
   d. Return to previous rate and variability.

4. Recovery with residual (sequence may vary):
   a. Decelerations diminish.
   b. Baseline rises, variability decreases.
   c. Decelerations disappear.
   d. Return to (stable) higher baseline and decreased variability.

5. Recovery from prolonged deceleration:
   a. Similar to above, but in addition:
   b. Late decelerations during recovery.

6. Deterioration—late decelerations:
   a. Decelerations increase.
   b. Baseline rises, variability decreases.
   c. Decelerations broader, smoother.

d. Variability absent.
e. Prolonged decelerations.
f. Unstable baseline, bradycardia, death.
7. Deterioration—variable decelerations:
   a. Amplitude increases.
   b. Baseline rises, variability decreases.
   c. "Shoulders" become exaggerated, peaked.
   d. Decelerations become smoother.
   e. Variability disappears.
   f. "Overshoot" pattern develops.
   g. Decelerations become longer.
   h. Unstable baseline, bradycardia, death.
8. Deterioration—prolonged decelerations:
   a. Rate returns toward previous baseline:
      1. May develop tachycardia, decreased variability. Decelerations repeat.
      2. New deceleration prevents return to baseline. Variability absent.
   b. Sustained low rate:
      1. If nodal rhythm—rate turns down.
      2. Loss of variability, unstable rate.

B. Principles of EFM interpretation.
1. Fetus always attempts to maintain stable baseline.
2. Baseline variability reflects fetal reserve.
3. Deceleration waveform reflects mechanism:
   a. Late decelerations—impaired uterine blood flow.
   b. Variable decelerations:
      1st stage—impaired umbilical blood flow.
      2nd stage—impaired cranial blood flow.
   c. Prolonged decelerations—several mechanisms.
4. Classifying decelerations in terms of amplitude, duration is of little practical value. Duration and amplitude of decelerations not reliable indicators of fetal insult.
5. Asphyxial decelerations elicit compensatory tachycardia and decreased variability whose duration are proportional to the insult.
6. Decelerations that "return slowly to baseline" but do not exceed the previous baseline rate do not represent an asphyxial insult. Assumes normal variability and absent tachycardia.

C. Principles of treatment.
1. Eliminate fetal nondistress—decelerations not all "steps on the road to death."
2. In most instances, fetal distress results from impaired uterine or umbilical blood flow.

3. Improve uterine blood flow:
   a. Minimize maternal hypotension.
   b. Avoid supine position.
   c. Reduce uterine contractions: decrease oxytocin, tocolysis.
4. Improve umbilical blood flow:
   a. Alter maternal position:
      Supine—lateral.
      Trendelenburg—knee-chest.
   b. Vaginal examination—search for cord.
   c. Elevate presenting part.
   d. Correct oligohydramnios—amnioinfusion.
   e. Stop pushing.
   f. Tocolysis.
5. Enhance maternal/fetal oxygen:
   a. Administer oxygen by tight face mask.
   b. Remove oxygen when recovery complete—may mask late decelerations.
   c. Glucose and bicarbonate inappropriate.
6. Restrict potentially compromising techniques (e.g., regional block, oxytocin, etc.) to the demonstrably normal fetus.
7. Assure that vaginal bleeding is not of fetal origin.

D. Therapy of variable decelerations.
1. Improve umbilical blood flow.
2. Oxygen—but not primary approach.

E. Therapy of late decelerations.
1. Improve uterine blood flow.
2. Oxygen—remove after recovery.

F. Therapy of prolonged decelerations.
1. Attempt correction as for variable decelerations:
   a. If good variability—anticipate recovery.
   b. If poor variability—consider intervention if not recovering within 4 minutes.
   c. Recovery likely with rising rate, increasing variability.
2. If pattern recovers—management philosophies:
   a. With obvious etiology (e.g., epidural): avoid the problem.
   b. With no obvious etiology—may intervene after second episode.
   c. Alternatively, may regard each episode as isolated incident—provided that recovery is complete.

G. Therapy of bradycardia—baseline <110 bpm.
1. Normal variability without decelerations:
   a. Normal fetus.
   b. Normal mother (MHR), dead fetus.
   c. Normal MHR pattern: accelerations with UC.

2. Absent variability without decelerations:
   a. Severely asphyxiated fetus, preterminal.
   b. Congenital heart block-diagnosis:
      Fetal ECG, ultrasound.
   c. Maternal collagen disease, CMV.

H. Principles of intervention.
1. Indications:
   a. Maternal.
   b. Fetal.
   c. Obstetrical.
   d. Other.
2. Fetal indication for intervention: non-remediable fetal distress.
3. Time to intervention:
   a. Optimal time not definable.
   b. Pattern recoverable—wait indefinitely.
   c. If not remediable: intervene safely, expeditiously.
4. Clues to recoverability:
   a. Cannot define with auscultation.
   b. Need continuous monitoring.
   c. Recover likely:
      Previously normal pattern.
      Demonstrable insult.
      Rate and variability return.
   d. Recovery unlikely:
      Sustained decelerations.
      Failed maneuvers.
      Absent baseline variability.
      Tachycardia or bradycardia.
      Variable decelerations with overshoot.
      Unstable rate, sinusoidal pattern.
5. Attempt intrauterine resuscitation—even when baby "deliverable."
6. No pattern "so ominous" that therapy not indicated.

C. Reapply monitor.
1. Unusual contractions, pain.
2. Ruptured membranes.
3. Return from bathroom.
4. Second stage/transition.
5. Medication/stimulation.

FETAL MONITORING UPON ADMISSION

A. Preliminary recording—normal criteria:
1. Stable heart rate.
2. Average variability—accelerations.
3. Absent decelerations with contractions.
B. Response.
1. If all criteria met—discontinue.
2. If abnormal—continue.

TRACINGS

TRACING: 01

CLINICAL: Normal pregnancy.

WEEKS: Term

BASELINE RATE: 140

STV: Decreased to average.

LTV: Average.

DECELERATIONS: None.

ACCELERATIONS: Variable, sporadic, prolonged.

UC: Irregular—early labor, oxytocin *(lower panel).*

OUTCOME: Normal term pregnancy.

COMMENT: This responsive fetus, at high station, reveals numerous accelerations with contractions. The appearance of the sinusoidal type pattern, at 8M and beyond, reflects prior administration of a narcotic analgesic. In the presence of accelerations, normal variability elsewhere, and the patient's history, this pattern carries no ominous connotation. Notice the narrow-ranged beat-to-beat arrhythmia (bigeminy) between 17M–20M and 23M–25M. These changes, sometimes artifactual, are occasionally seen with sympathomimetic drugs and "-caine" anesthetics administered via epidural (as here) or paracervical block—this is a benign response. The exaggerated acceleration after 25M represents a response to a pelvic examination and is of no consequence considering the rapid return to baseline and resumption of variability.

The frequent contractions reasonably preclude the restarting of the oxytocin at 21M. The appearance of hyperstimulation beginning at 25M should come as no surprise. Running the oxytocin at a very low, constant rate may improve the contraction pattern as well as avoid excessive stimulation.

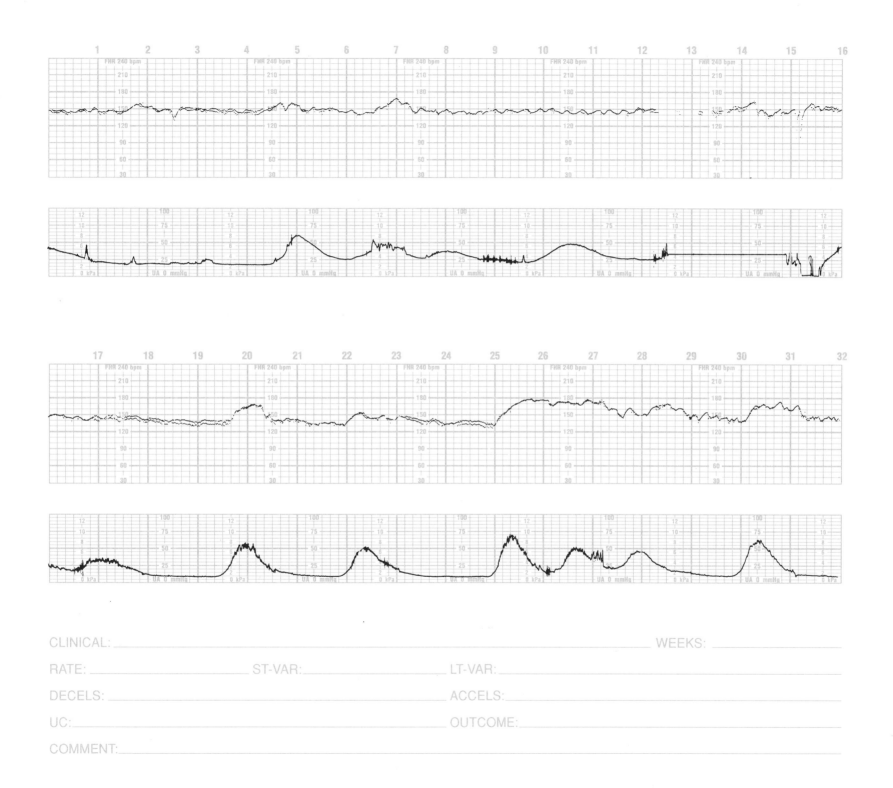

CLINICAL: _____ WEEKS: _____

RATE: _____ ST-VAR: _____ LT-VAR: _____

DECELS: _____ ACCELS: _____

UC: _____ OUTCOME: _____

COMMENT: _____

TRACING: 02

CLINICAL: Uneventful prenatal course.

WEEKS: 40

BASELINE RATE: 150–160

STV: Average.

LTV: Average.

DECELERATIONS: None.

ACCELERATIONS: Coalesced.

UC: Early labor.

OUTCOME: Apgar scores, 9/9; uneventful neonatal course.

COMMENT: This tracing illustrates state changes in the fetus during early labor in a very excitable mother. Notice the three distinct FHR patterns in the *top panel*. In the first 5 minutes the pattern is characterized by diminished short- and long-term variability. This probably represents quiet sleep. From 5M to 12M, the short- and long-term variability increases and the rate decreases. This likely represents fetal breathing, but there are no obvious accelerations. From 12M to 16M the tracing becomes reactive with normal variability, obvious accelerations, and, pre- sumably, fetal movement. This continuum certainly represents the different state changes within the fetus. They are not infre- quently seen early in labor, irrespective of contractions. The ap- parent deceleration at 22M is simply a return to the baseline rate for that state and is not dissimilar from the shallow trough at 7M, which anticipates the accelerations. Notice that the greater the variability the lower the baseline heart rate. Notice also the changes in the mother's (hyper)ventilation pattern as reflected on the uterine contraction channel. This is a reassuring tracing.

22

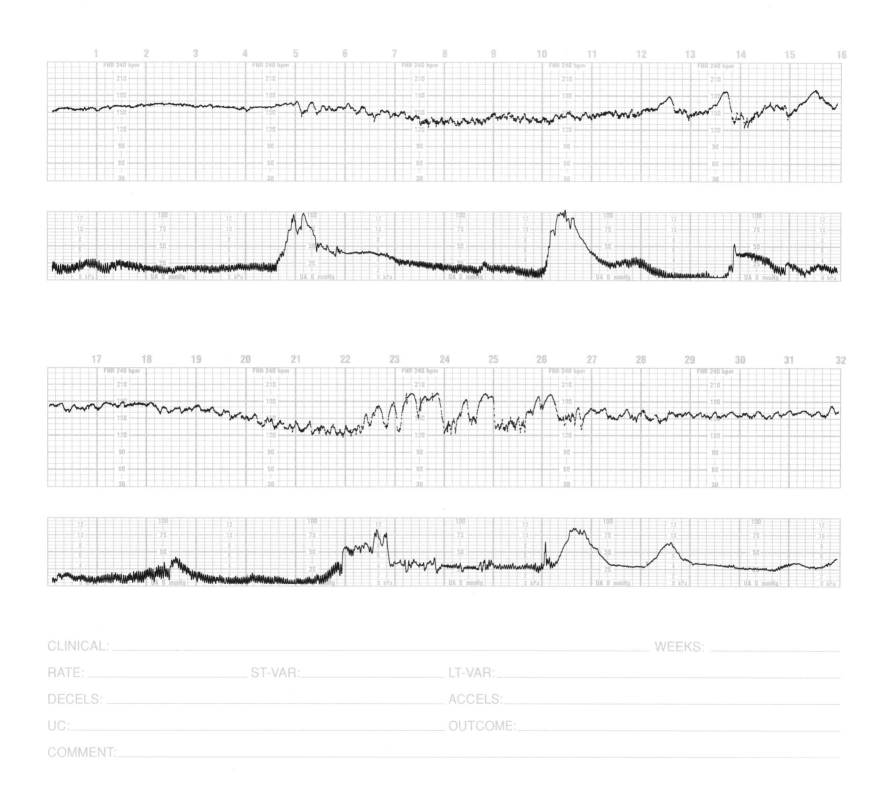

CLINICAL: _____   WEEKS: _____

RATE: _____   ST-VAR: _____   LT-VAR: _____

DECELS: _____   ACCELS: _____

UC: _____   OUTCOME: _____

COMMENT: _____

TRACING: 03

CLINICAL: Normal pregnancy, high station.

WEEKS: 40

BASELINE RATE: A: 120. B: 150.

STV: Average.

LTV: Average.

DECELERATIONS: None.

ACCELERATIONS: Sporadic.

UC: A: Sporadic. B: Oxytocin.

OUTCOME: Normal, cesarean section, failure of descent.

COMMENT: These tracings were obtained several hours apart. The *upper panel,* obtained with an ultrasound transducer, reveals abundant accelerations, a stable baseline rate and apparently normal variability. The *lower panel,* obtained with a direct scalp electrode on a high head, continues to reveal accelerations during and between contractions. In the interim between the *upper* and *lower panels,* the patient has received narcotics, epidural anesthesia, and oxytocin. The analgesics have diminished the variability of the baseline between accelerations but, if anything, have increased their frequency.

These accelerations are probably associated with fetal movement. Fetal reactivity may persist into early or mid-labor despite the administration of analgesia. In the *lower panel,* note the regular contractions and the regular maternal breathing pattern.

A

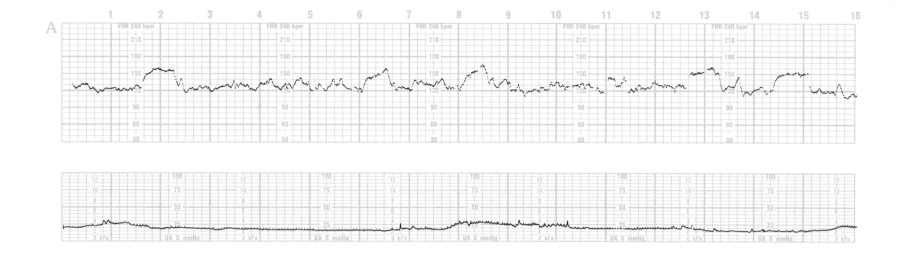

B

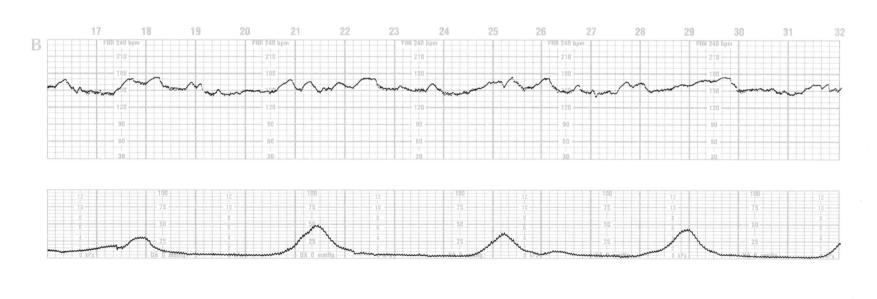

CLINICAL: _____ WEEKS: _____

RATE: _____ ST-VAR: _____ LT-VAR: _____

DECELS: _____ ACCELS: _____

UC: _____ OUTCOME: _____

COMMENT: _____

TRACING: 04

CLINICAL: Normal pregnancy, early labor.

WEEKS: 37

BASELINE RATE: 150

STV: Average, decreased.

LTV: Average.

DECELERATIONS: Occasional, variable.

ACCELERATIONS: Numerous, sporadic, coalescence (9M−13M).

UC: Irregular, early labor.

OUTCOME: Normal.

COMMENT: This tracing reveals some features of benign accelerations. While the baseline variability is somewhat diminished (possibly the *effect of medication*) some event at 8M+, perhaps a pelvic examination, promotes a sustained acceleration lasting about 5 minutes. Notice the "scalloped" appearance of these coalesced accelerations, and the suggestion of small decelerations with overshoot that they create. This pattern of accelerations is a normal response.

In the *lower panel,* the apparent decelerations at 18M, 20M, and 22M really represent an "undershooting" of the baseline following an acceleration (the lambda pattern); they are not decelerations. This is a benign pattern irrespective of the timing, amplitude, or duration of the lambda pattern.

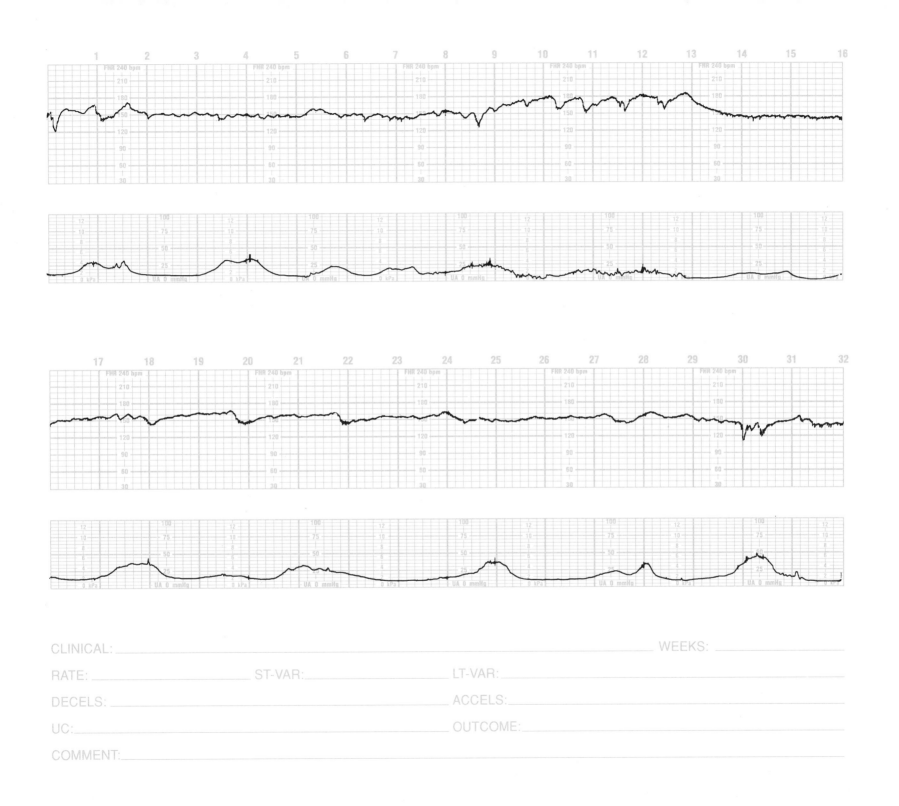

TRACING: 05

CLINICAL: Normal pregnancy, breech presentation.

WEEKS: 38

BASELINE RATE: 150–160

STV: Average.

LTV: Average.

DECELERATIONS: None.

ACCELERATIONS: Sporadic, exaggerated.

UC: Active labor.

OUTCOME: Normal.

COMMENT: This otherwise unremarkable tracing becomes dramatic in the lower panel with the appearance of exaggerated accelerations exceeding 50 bpm in amplitude. Generally, they represent normal variants, especially when accompanied by normal variability and stable baseline rates. These accelerations generally appear early in labor with the head high or with nonvertex presentation, as in this case. Maternal anxiety (or drug addiction) may contribute to the size of the accelerations. Note the compulsive maternal breathing efforts during contractions.

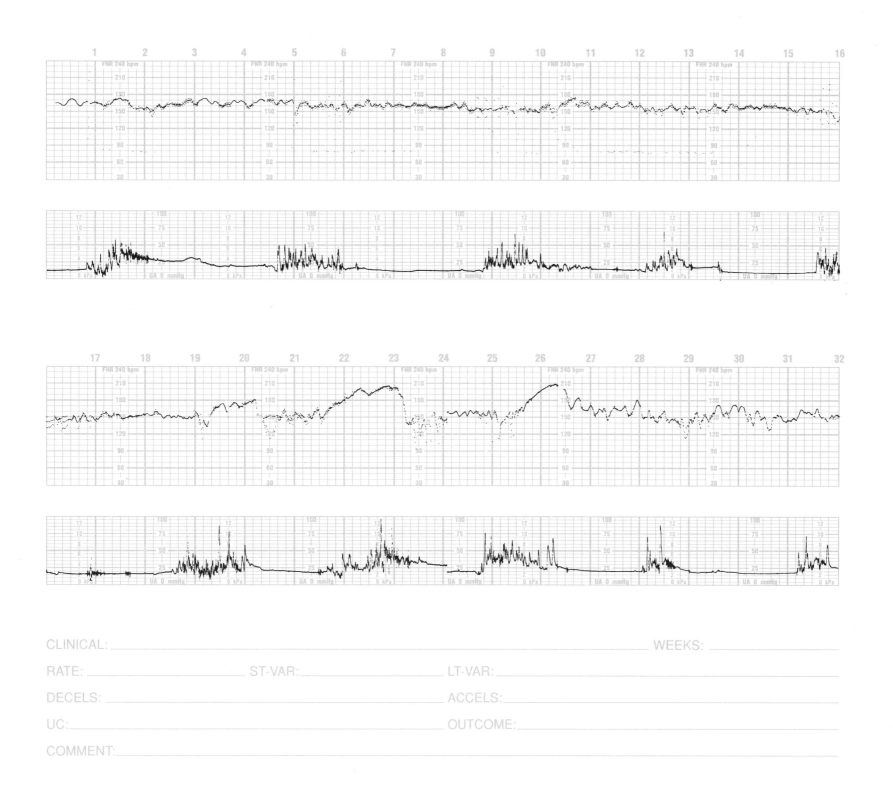

CLINICAL: _____ WEEKS: _____

RATE: _____ ST-VAR: _____ LT-VAR: _____

DECELS: _____ ACCELS: _____

UC: _____ OUTCOME: _____

COMMENT: _____

TRACING: 06

CLINICAL: Uneventful course, transverse lie, funic presentation.

WEEKS: 40

BASELINE RATE: 125

STV: Average.

LTV: Average.

DECELERATIONS: Variable (see text).

ACCELERATIONS: Uniform, sporadic.

UC: Every 3 minutes.

OUTCOME: Apgar scores, 8/9; uneventful neonatal course.

COMMENT: This tracing was recorded at 1 cm/minute from a term fetus with a transverse lie and funic (cord) presentation. Under experimental conditions, with the patient on the operating table prepared for cesarean section, the umbilical cord was clamped between the examiner's fingers for 6 seconds. A similar episode is shown at 17M. These maneuvers produced transient variable decelerations with prompt, immediate recovery. Notice the characteristic accelerations with contractions, which are the hallmark of the nonvertex presentation. Immediately after the tracing was taken, the patient underwent cesarean section with delivery of a normal fetus.

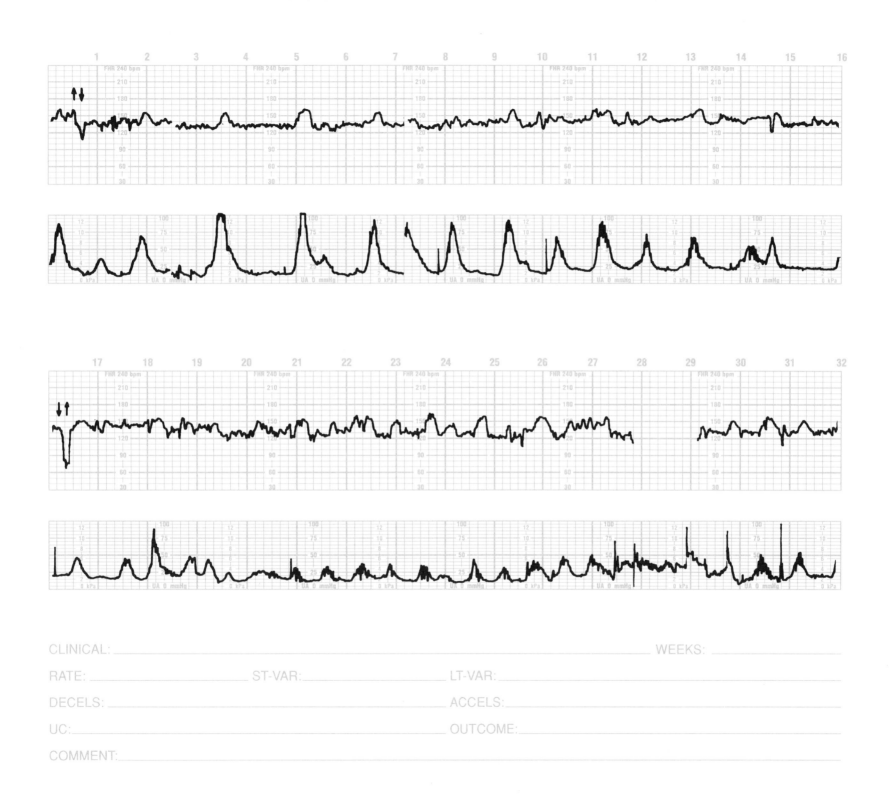

CLINICAL: _____ WEEKS: _____

RATE: _____ ST-VAR: _____ LT-VAR: _____

DECELS: _____ ACCELS: _____

UC: _____ OUTCOME: _____

COMMENT: _____

TRACING: 07

CLINICAL: Normal pregnancy.

WEEKS: Term

BASELINE RATE: 130–140

STV: Average.

LTV: Average.

DECELERATIONS: None!

ACCELERATIONS: Sporadic, coalescence.

UC: Early labor.

OUTCOME: Normal.

COMMENT: This tracing illustrates several features of fetal accelerations in the resilient fetus. Accelerations may be isolated, coupled, or coalesced. Sporadic accelerations associated with fetal movement tend to be angular, with a more sweeping ascent and prompt return to baseline—often with a little deceleration at the end (the so-called lambda pattern). Accelerations with contractions (high-station, nonvertex presentations, atropine) tend to be more uniform. Either may be punctuated with a brief, variable deceleration that is insignificant. When accelerations coalesce, they may simulate tachycardia (15M) or be "scalloped" (13M). The *lower panel* represents an exaggerated "scallop" pattern, probably associated with fetal sucking and decreased fetal movement. Note the resemblance here to frequent, small, variable decelerations with overshoot. During an acceleration, variability is always decreased. This is a benign pattern.

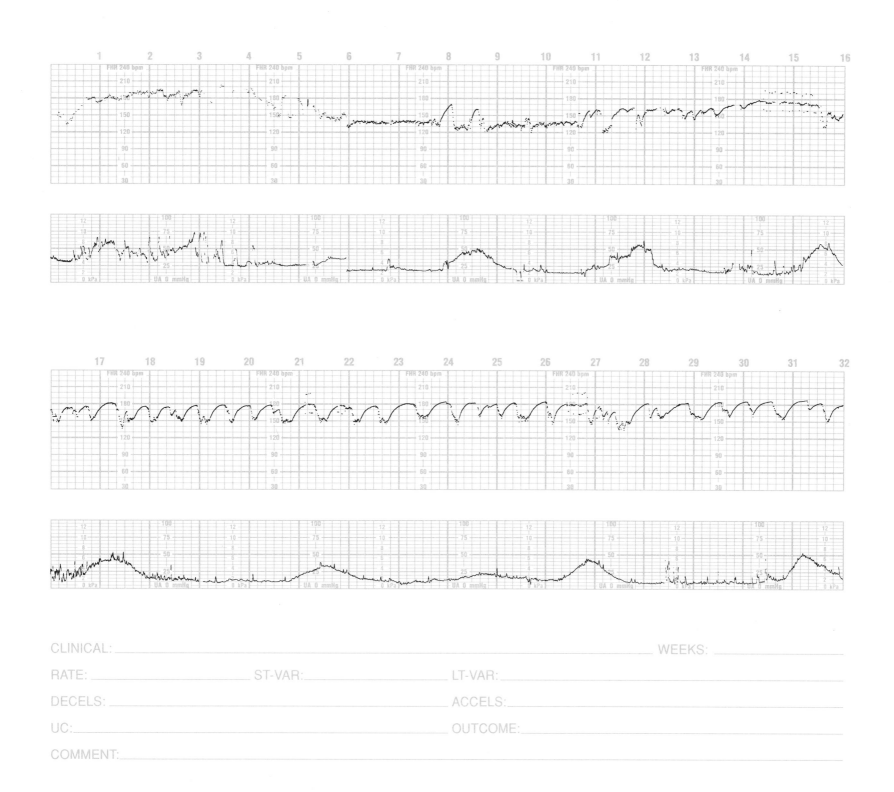

CLINICAL: _____ WEEKS: _____

RATE: _____ ST-VAR: _____ LT-VAR: _____

DECELS: _____ ACCELS: _____

UC: _____ OUTCOME: _____

COMMENT: _____

TRACING: 08

CLINICAL: Multipara, uneventful pregnancy.

WEEKS: 38

BASELINE RATE: 155

STV: Decreased.

LTV: Decreased.

DECELERATIONS: Early.

ACCELERATIONS: Uniform.

UC: Regular, oxytocin effect.

OUTCOME: Apgar scores, 8/9; uneventful neonatal course.

COMMENT: This tracing demonstrates the effects of station and ruptured membranes on fetal heart rate (FHR) patterns. The *top panel* was obtained early in labor with external transducers and reveals average variability and unequivocal accelerations with contractions. The accelerations tend to be irregular; they are occasionally followed by small decelerations (lambda pattern). In the *lower panel* the diminished variability and regular oscillations (sinusoidal pattern) between accelerations is a result of administration of a narcotic to the mother. When membranes rupture or the fetus gains station, the accelerations disappear and are replaced by recurrent, small, early decelerations. The regular amplitude and interval of the uterine contractions suggest oxytocin administration. This is a reassuring tracing.

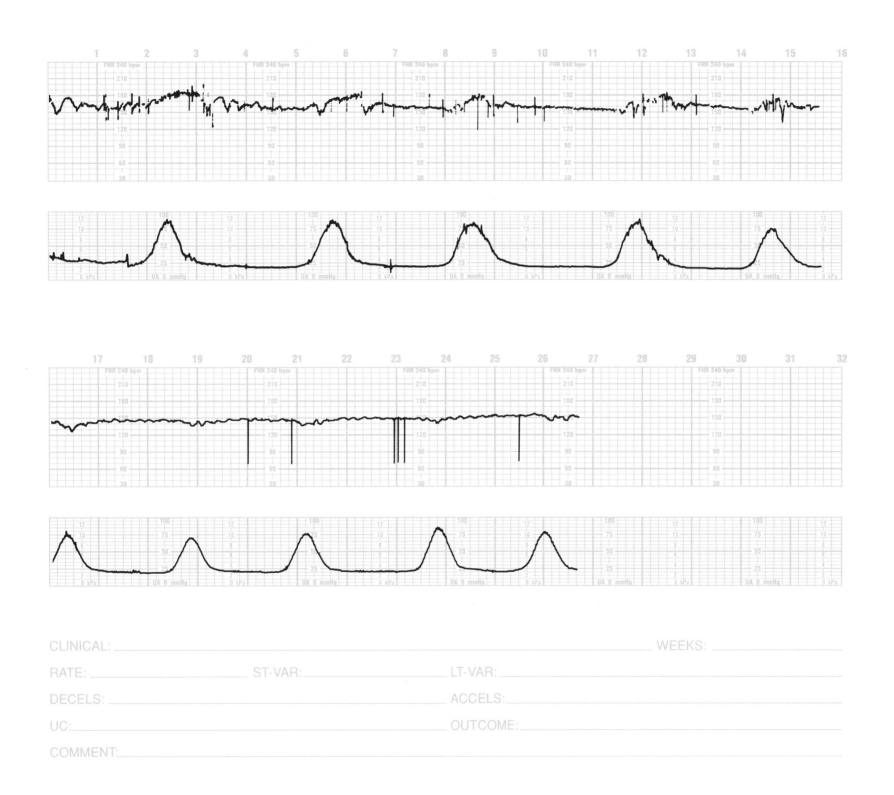

TRACING: 09

CLINICAL: Uneventful prenatal course.

WEEKS: 39

BASELINE RATE: 135

STV: Average.

LTV: Average.

DECELERATIONS: Variable.

ACCELERATIONS: Variable ("shoulders").

UC: Effect of position change.

OUTCOME: Apgar scores, 9/9; uneventful neonatal course.

COMMENT: This tracing illustrates the differences in uterine activity patterns in the supine and lateral positions. For the *upper tracing,* the patient is in the supine position; in the *lower panel* the patient has been moved to the left lateral position. In the supine position, contractions are of lower amplitude and higher frequency compared with the lateral position. In this case, the patient's placement in the lateral position is accompanied by changes in both FHR pattern and uterine activity. The baseline variability increases and variable decelerations appear in association with higher amplitude but less frequent contractions. Nevertheless, this tracing is quite reassuring, as baseline variability and accelerations are maintained satisfactorily throughout.

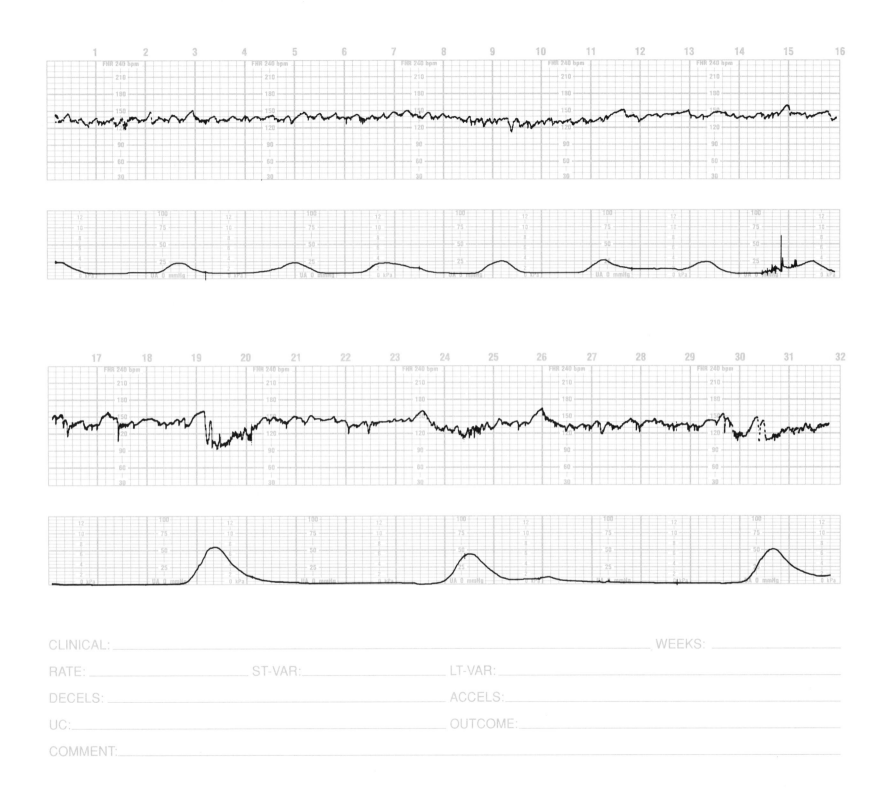

TRACING: 10

CLINICAL: Uneventful prenatal course.

WEEKS: 39

BASELINE RATE: 155

STV: Average to decreased.

LTV: Average.

DECELERATIONS: Variable.

ACCELERATIONS: Variable ("shoulders").

UC: Oxytocin.

OUTCOME: Apgar scores, 7/9; uneventful neonatal course.

COMMENT: This tracing illustrates changes in uterine activity following paracervical block. In early labor, contractions tend to be irregular in amplitude, duration, and interval. Indeed, the earlier in labor that analgesics or anesthetic agents are administered, the more likely they diminish uterine activity and prolong labor. Local anesthetic agents, irrespective of injection site, may either increase, decrease, or have no effect on uterine activity. In this tracing, paracervical block at 17M produces a dramatic decrease in the frequency of uterine contractions despite the continuing oxytocin infusion. The frequent, variable decelerations are associated with the low station and the manipulations required to inject the anesthetic. The apparent deceleration (at 15M) does not qualify as a late deceleration, as it is unassociated with similar decelerations elsewhere. Further, it is anticipated by several accelerations.

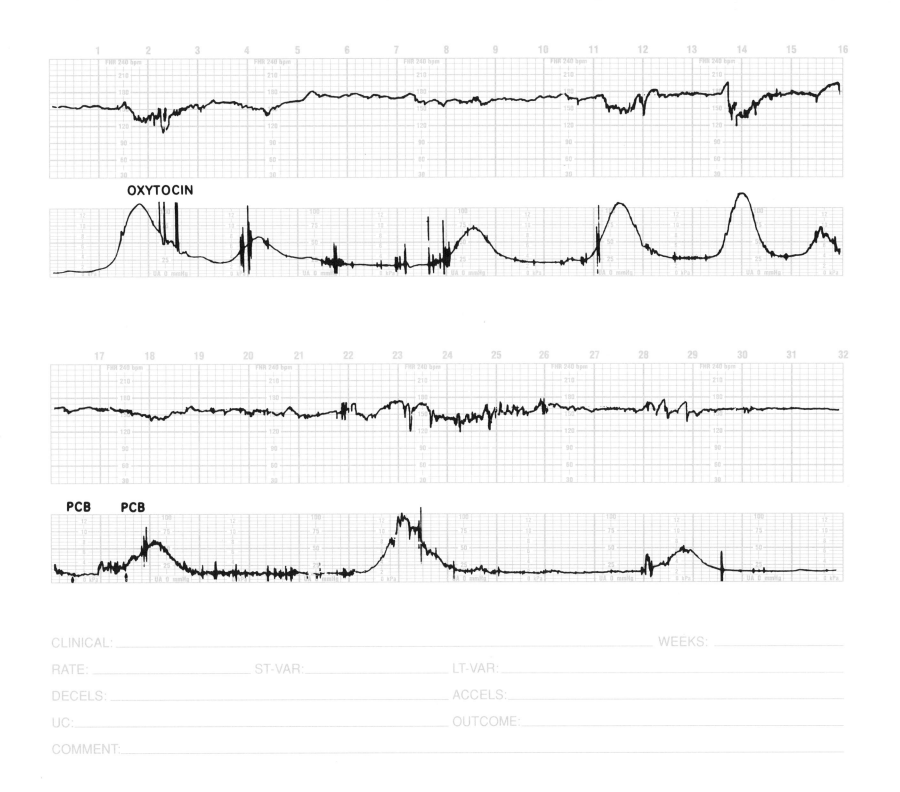

OXYTOCIN

PCB   PCB

CLINICAL:_____   WEEKS:_____

RATE:_____   ST-VAR:_____   LT-VAR:_____

DECELS:_____   ACCELS:_____

UC:_____   OUTCOME:_____

COMMENT:_____

TRACING: 11

CLINICAL: Both: uneventful prenatal course.

WEEKS: A: 41. B: 39.

BASELINE RATE: A: 170. B: 130.

STV: A: Decreased. B: Average.

LTV: A: Decreased. B: Average.

DECELERATIONS: Both: none.

ACCELERATIONS: Both: none.

UC: A: Infrequent, second stage. B: Regular.

OUTCOME: Both: Apgar scores, 8/9; uneventful neonatal course.

COMMENT: The *upper* and *lower panels* represent different fetuses. Alterations in the FHR pattern in the second stage of labor are quite common and increase during bearing-down efforts. With infrequent contractions the patterns may be neither dramatic nor consistent, and classification of these FHR changes will not be satisfying. In the *upper panel,* the decelerations begin at different times and show different characteristics. One must resist the temptation to call the first one a late deceleration. Late decelerations must be repetitive, uniform, and, in any given sequence, proportional in amplitude and duration to the amplitude and duration of the underlying contraction. It *seems* far more appropriate to refer to these patterns simply as "increased variability associated with contractions (pushing)." The diminution in variability between these episodes is a function of administration of a narcotic to the mother.

In the *lower panel,* the appearance of regular oscillations in the baseline invites the designation "sinusoidal pattern." In this instance, the somewhat irregular oscillations tend to be peaked and seem to contain short-term variability. Such patterns may be seen with the normal rest-activity cycles in the healthy fetus. Indeed, other areas of the tracing reveal normal reactivity. In the presence of variability or reactivity, sinusoidal features may be dismissed. True sinusoidal patterns, even those developing after the administration of narcotics, tend to be smoother and less angular, and are associated with decreased baseline variability.

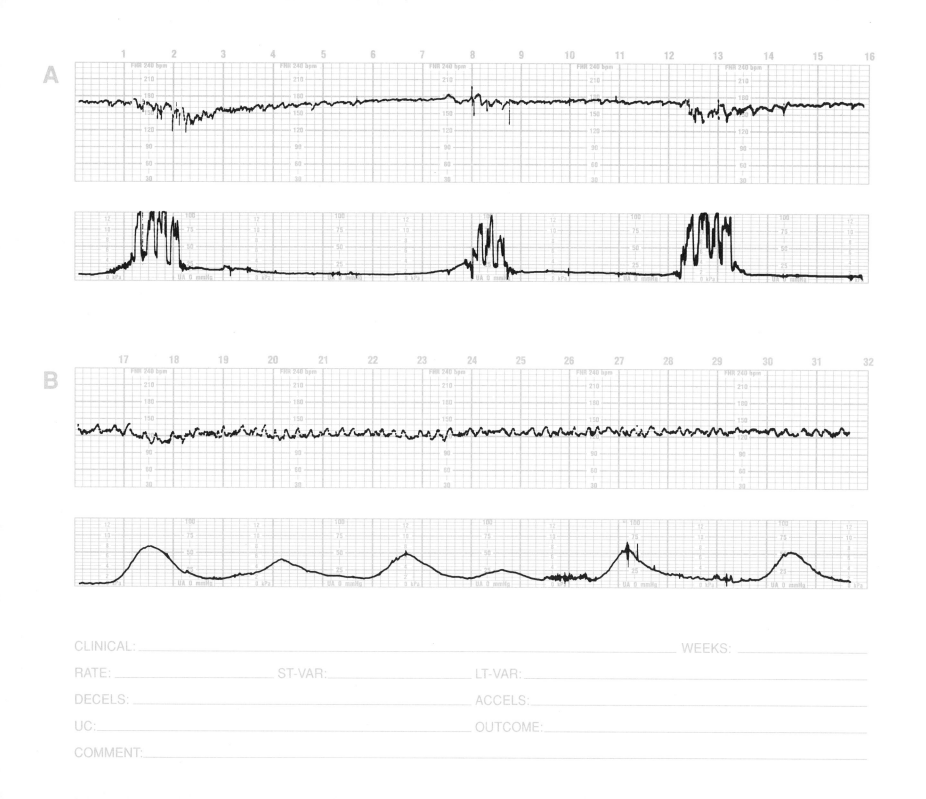

CLINICAL: _____ WEEKS: _____

RATE: _____ ST-VAR: _____ LT-VAR: _____

DECELS: _____ ACCELS: _____

UC: _____ OUTCOME: _____

COMMENT: _____

TRACING: 12

CLINICAL: Uneventful pregnancy.

WEEKS: 41

BASELINE RATE: 130–150

STV: Average.

LTV: Average.

DECELERATIONS: Variable.

ACCELERATIONS: Uniform, variable ("shoulders").

UC: Early labor, irregular in amplitude and interval.

OUTCOME: Uneventful neonatal course.

COMMENT: This tracing illustrates the benefits of hydrating the patient and maintaining her in a lateral position prior to the administration of epidural anesthesia. There are occasional, variable decelerations but late decelerations are absent despite the drop in blood pressure at 20M and the increase in uterine activity from the epidural block. Although there is no significant impact on the baseline rate, there is some diminution in the short-term (but not long-term) variability in the lower panel. This is a pharmacological effect of systemic absorption of local anesthetic by the mother and subsequent transplacental passage to the fetus. This is a reassuring tracing.

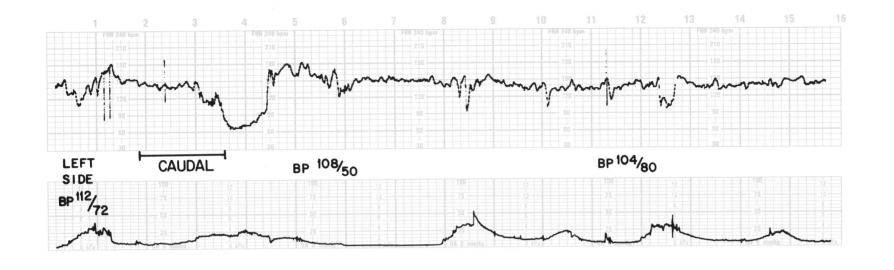

LEFT
SIDE

CAUDAL

BP 108/50

BP 104/80

BP 112/72

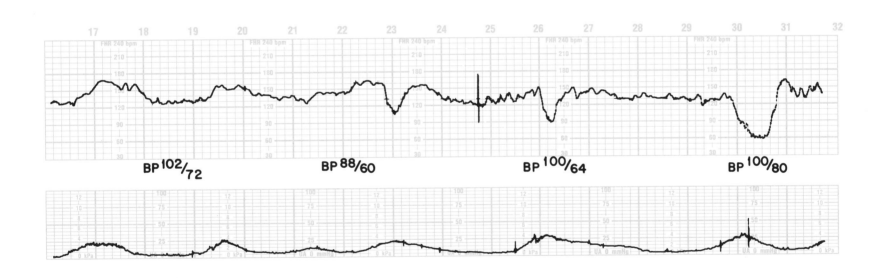

BP 102/72

BP 88/60

BP 100/64

BP 100/80

TRACING: 13

CLINICAL: Normal term pregnancy.

WEEKS: Term

BASELINE RATE: 130–140

STV: Average.

LTV: Average, increased.

DECELERATIONS: Variable.

ACCELERATIONS: Variable.

UC: Oxytocin *(lower tracing).*

OUTCOME: Normal.

COMMENT: In this variant of a normal pattern there are frequent, small, abrupt decelerations that subscribe to no consistent pattern, but occasionally mimic variable decelerations with overshoot. These somewhat chaotic patterns tend to be seen early in labor and sometimes after episodes of anxiety in the mother. While the fetus may be active, typical accelerations are not seen. Contractions seem to exaggerate these features. While these patterns imply no adverse condition in the fetus, the mechanism for their production is not clear.

The pattern changes dramatically in the *lower panel,* obtained about 1 hour later. Here, oxytocin infusion induces regular uterine contractions. In addition, a narcotic, administered to relieve the mother's pain during contractions, also relieves any pain the fetus might be feeling. As a result, the earlier chaotic pattern in the fetal tracing is replaced by regular, predictable oscillations (sinusoidal pattern) that are interrupted by mild (early or variable) decelerations. Despite their dramatic differences, these patterns are quite benign and require no intervention.

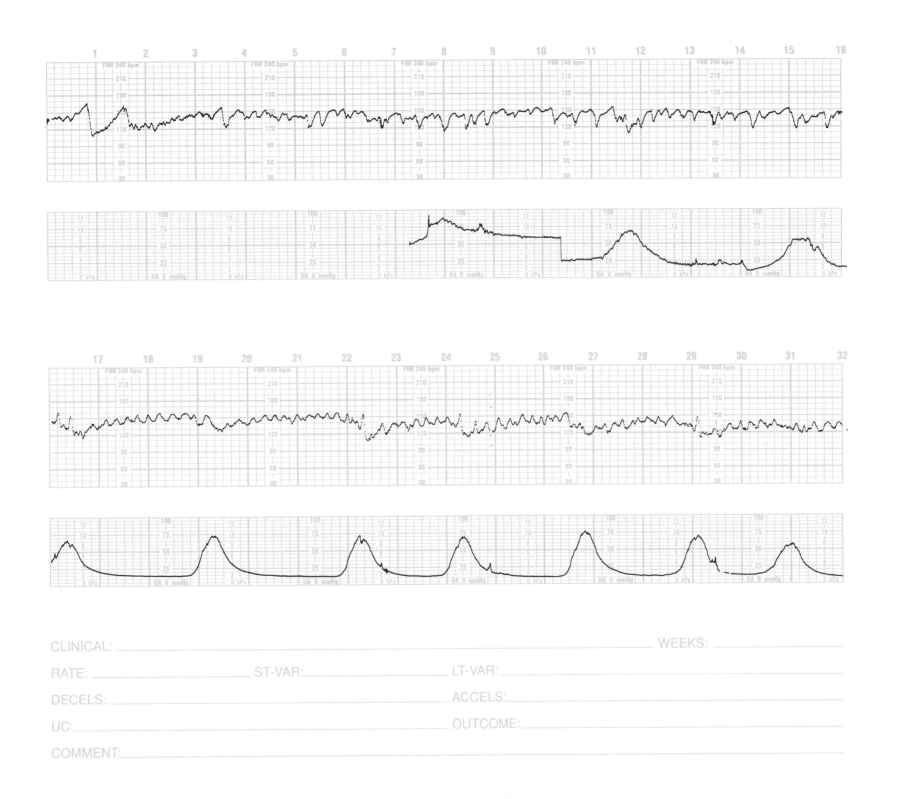

CLINICAL: _____ WEEKS: _____

RATE: _____ ST-VAR: _____ LT-VAR: _____

DECELS: _____ ACCELS: _____

UC: _____ OUTCOME: _____

COMMENT: _____

TRACING: 14

CLINICAL: Normal pregnancy, occiput anterior.

WEEKS: Both: term.

BASELINE RATE: A: 130. B: 110–120.

STV: A: Average, increased. B: Decreased.

LTV: A: Average. B: Decreased.

DECELERATIONS: A: Early, mild variable. B: Absent.

ACCELERATIONS: A: Sporadic. B: Absent.

UC: Both: Late labor, regular contractions on oxytocin.

OUTCOME: Both: Normal.

COMMENT: These tracings illustrate greater and lesser variability and greater and lesser artifact. The *upper tracing* was obtained during the second stage of labor with the patient receiving oxytocin stimulation under epidural anesthesia (observe the quiet UC recording between contractions). Between contractions, the artifact-free FHR pattern shows considerable variability and some accelerations at 3M, 8M, 10M, and elsewhere. During contractions, the tracing reveals considerable artifact associated with the mother's bearing-down efforts and probably some small variable decelerations. While the only certain way to prove that these abrupt excursions during the contractions are artifact and not arrhythmia is to obtain a fetal ECG, the inference that these are artifact is compelling. These abrupt excursions appear only during expulsive efforts and are strictly limited to the period of contractions (except for the single spike at 15M). The pattern reveals no real symmetry and the upper limit of the excursions is bounded only by the limitations of the recording pen. These excursions appear unrelated to the transient decelerations. In addition, the frequency of the excursions varies considerably, irrespective of the presence of decelerations (compare the changes at 8M and 10M). This is a normal second stage pattern in a term baby with occiput anterior and a high head.

The *lower panel* reflects a low, stable heart rate with decreased variability and occasional minimal accelerations. Between 16M and 23M the pattern reveals high-frequency (24/minute) and very low-amplitude oscillations. These changes appear to carry no ominous importance.

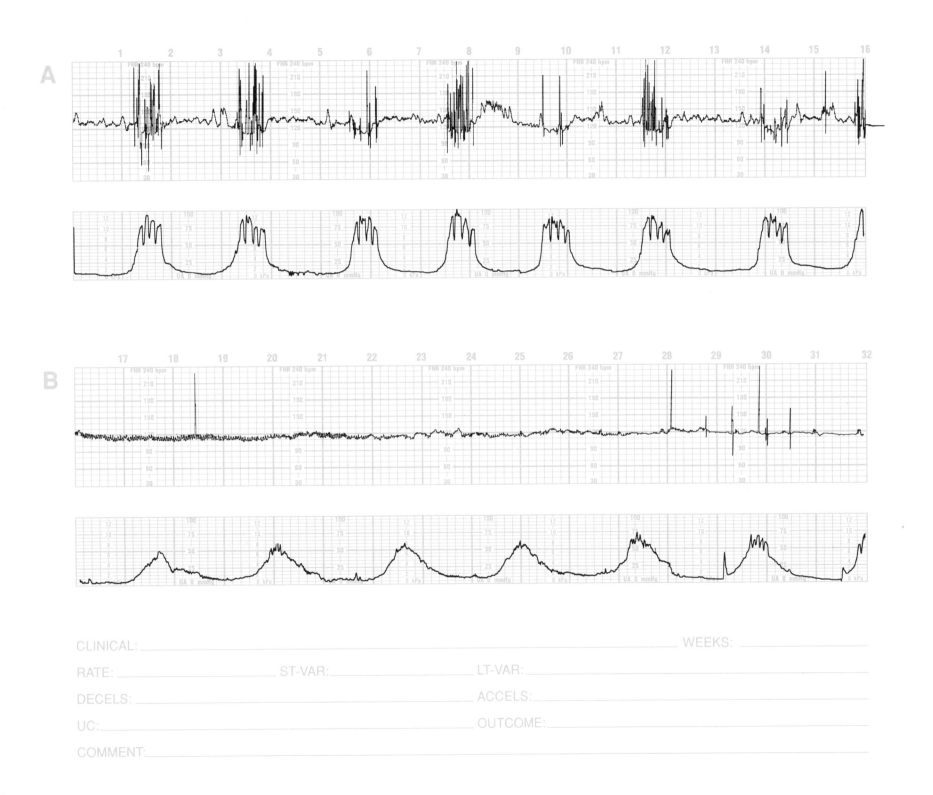

A

B

TRACING: 15

CLINICAL: Uneventful prenatal course.

WEEKS: 41

BASELINE RATE: 130

STV: Decreased.

LTV: Decreased.

DECELERATIONS: None.

ACCELERATIONS: None.

UC: Response to paracervical block, tachysystole.

OUTCOME: Apgar scores, 6/9; uneventful prenatal course.

COMMENT: This tracing illustrates some benign effects of paracervical block anesthesia (administered at 17M). Prior to administration of the block, the baby's heart rate is quite stable at 130 bpm but with diminished short-term variability. Sinusoidal undulations in the baseline reflect the previous administration of narcotic to the mother. The administration of the block and the manipulations associated with it produces a dramatic increase in the amount of variability and accelerations in the heart rate. There is also some increase in the frequency of uterine contrac- tions. The short-lived deceleration that begins at 27M recovers promptly and is unassociated with any further decelerations.

While paracervical block anesthesia is not widely used, it is an extraordinarily satisfying anesthesia in the first stage of labor. The procedure requires minimal dosages, injected at least 5 minutes apart, and careful attention to technique lest the drug be injected into the myometrium. Marcaine (bupivacaine) should not be used for paracervical blocks.

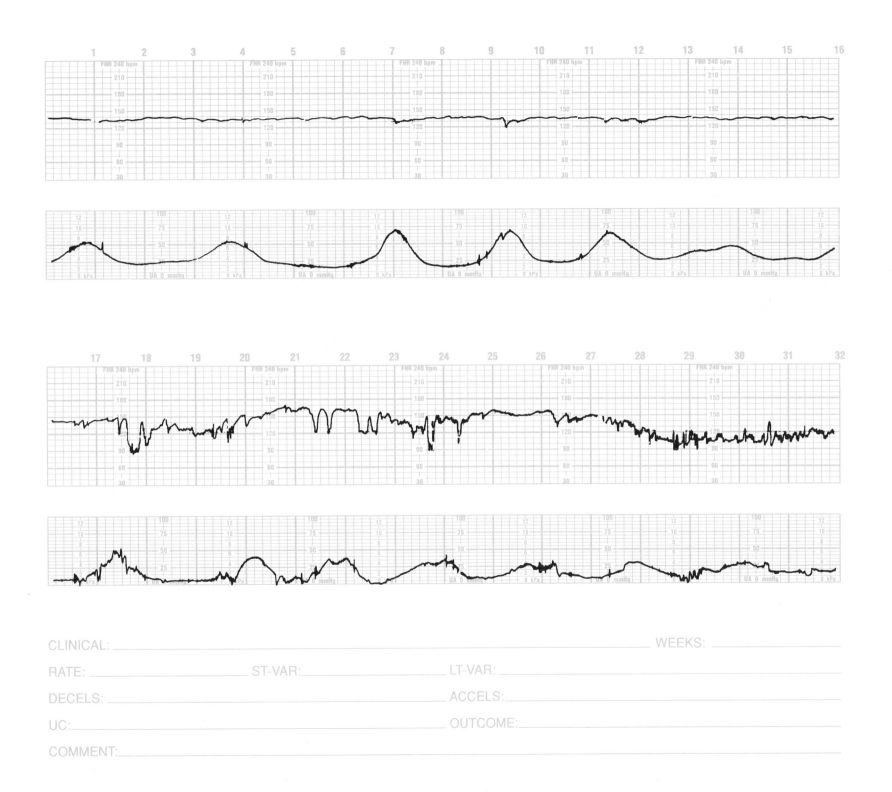

TRACING: 16

CLINICAL: Normal pregnancy.

WEEKS: Term

BASELINE RATE: 140

STV: Average to decreased.

LTV: Decreased.

DECELERATIONS: None.

ACCELERATIONS: None.

UC: Sporadic, occasional.

OUTCOME: Normal.

COMMENT: This tracing, obtained in early labor, reflects several effects of medication on the FHR pattern and uterine contractions. Narcotics decrease baseline variability as well as the frequency and angularity of the accelerations associated with fetal movement. Notice that the accelerations appear only with contractions, if at all, and that the accelerations arise from diminished variability. Although there is some variability at the beginning of the tracing, this diminishes considerably as a result of administration of the medication. In active labor, narcotics usually have little or no effect on uterine contractions. In early labor they may either depress uterine activity (as here) or occasionally exaggerate it. If this were a non-stress test the result would be non-reactive.

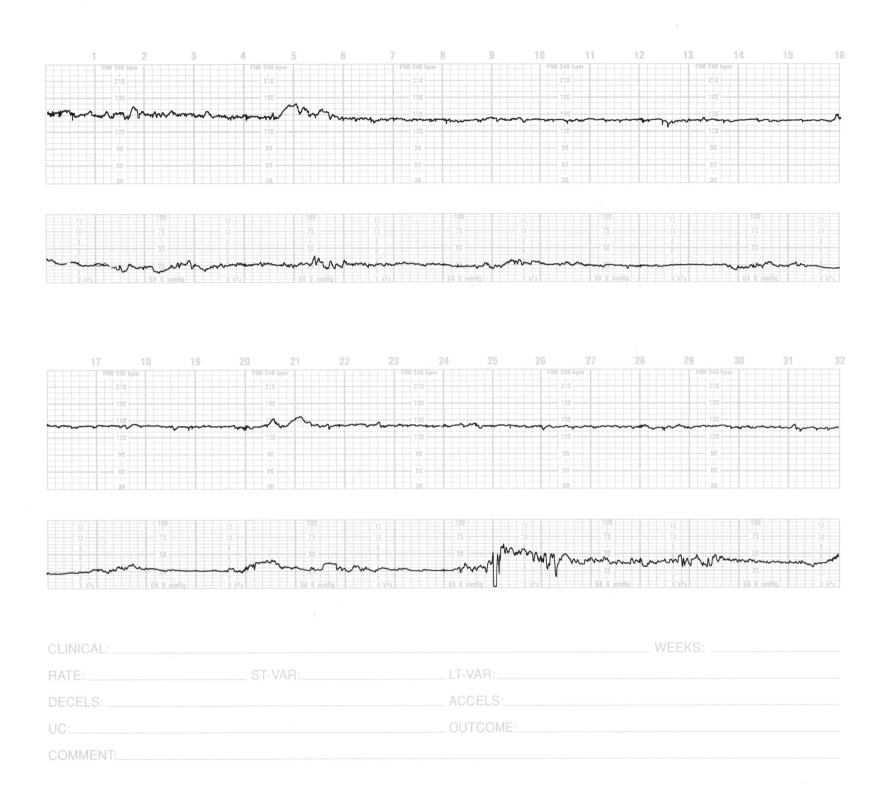

TRACING: 17

CLINICAL: Uneventful prenatal course.

WEEKS: 38

BASELINE RATE: 140–155

STV: Decreased.

LTV: Decreased.

DECELERATIONS: Absent.

ACCELERATIONS: Sporadic.

UC: Hypertonus, tachysystole.

OUTCOME: Apgar scores, 7/9; uneventful neonatal course.

COMMENT: This tracing illustrates the effect of paracervical block on uterine activity. Local anesthetic agents such as Xylocaine (lidocaine), Carbocaine (mepivacaine), and Marcaine (bupivacaine), all have the potential for increasing uterine activity irrespective of the route of administration. Indeed, the most consistent finding associated with "paracervical block bradycardia" is uterine hypertonus. In this case, the excessive uterine activity develops shortly after the administration of paracervical block at 20M and persists for the remainder of the tracing. Despite the excessive uterine activity there are no decelerations. The decreased short-term variability, the suggestion of (sinusoidal) oscillations induced by narcotics and the frequent contractions clearly antedate the administration of the block. The benign nature of the diminution in variability is reflected in the accelerations in the heart rate at 1M and again at 28M. The vertical spikes likely represent random, inconsistent artifact associated with the manipulation preceding the block and the attempt at scalp sampling at 26M.

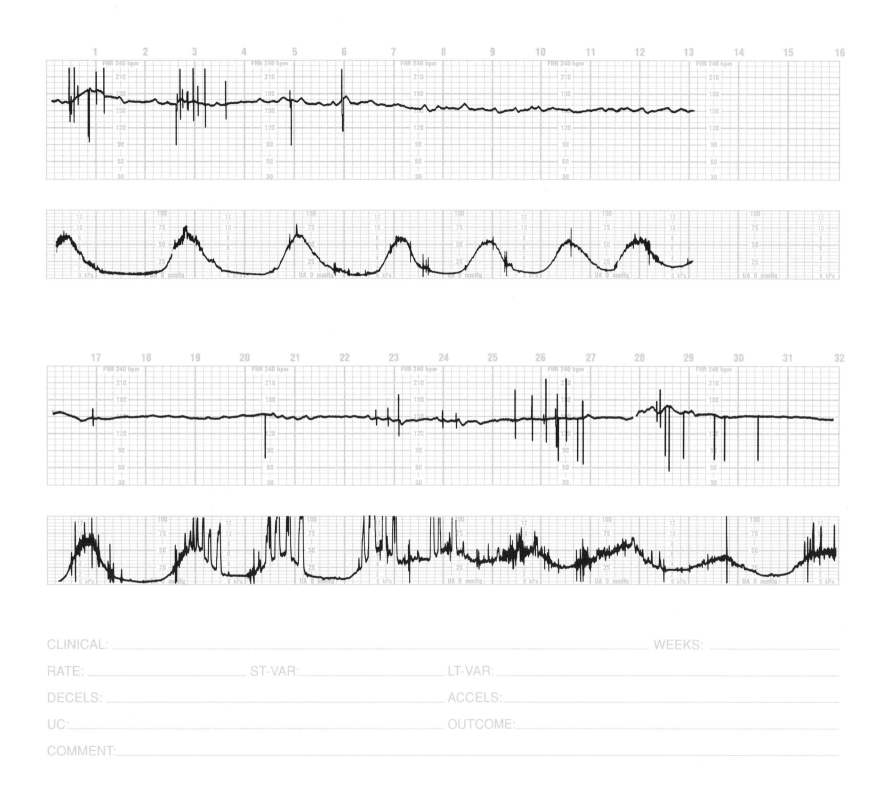

TRACING: 18

CLINICAL: Post-date pregnancy, nonreactive NST.

WEEKS: 43

BASELINE RATE: 120

STV: Probably decreased.

LTV: Decreased.

DECELERATIONS: None.

ACCELERATIONS: None.

UC: Sporadic (upper), oxytocin (lower).

OUTCOME: Congenital anomaly.

COMMENT: Though obtained by external transducers and containing considerable artifact, these tracings, obtained several hours apart, give the impression of markedly reduced variability, both short- and long-term. There is a remote possibility that these abrupt excursions might represent arrhythmia that is undetectable with an external device. With arrhythmia, however, the pattern tends to be more geometrically predictable and organized, even if the full excursions are not seen. The artifact-free areas at 23M, 25M, 27M, and, to a lesser extent, 18M could not be flatter nor the fetus less responsive to the effects of the frequent uterine contractions. Although several areas suggest accelerations or decelerations, these excursions are quite limited in amplitude, are associated with increased artifact, and correspond to no consistent pattern. Asphyxia is a most improbable cause of such tracings. The low, stable baseline reveals no significant or consistent decelerations or sinusoidal oscillations. The annotated and unannotated instances of fetal movement produce perhaps a single acceleration of minimal amplitude and a trailing deceleration (a lambda pattern). The differential diagnosis of this combination of decreased variability with fetal movement present includes prematurity, drug effect, neurologic handicap, or congenital anomaly.

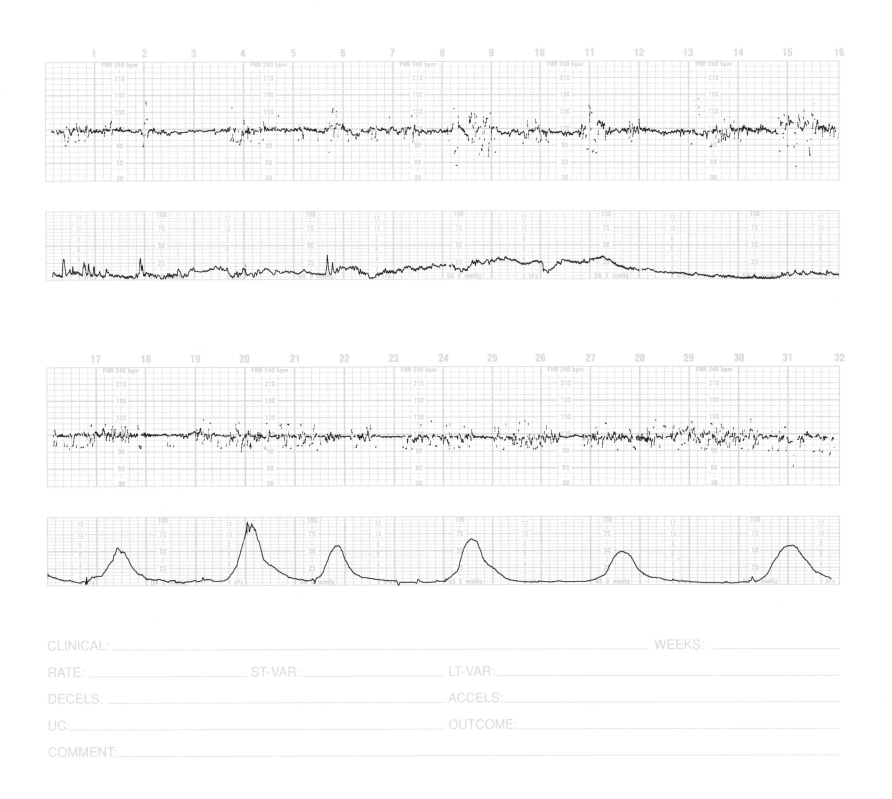

TRACING: 19

CLINICAL: Normal pregnancy, early labor.

WEEKS: 36

BASELINE RATE: 150

STV: Decreased, absent.

LTV: Decreased, absent.

DECELERATIONS: Unclassified, trivial.

ACCELERATIONS: Occasional, sporadic.

UC: Poorly recorded at first; regular, active labor.

OUTCOME: Normal infant.

COMMENT: This tracing beguiles us with diminished variability, which is made more obvious in the *upper panel* by the changeover from ultrasound transducer to direct fetal scalp electrode at 6M. The excursions between 6M and 7M represent artifact associated with the initial attachment of the electrode and stabilization of the fetal signal in the monitor, and do not constitute fetal arrhythmia. There are no decelerations in the *upper panel* but the frequency of contractions is minimal. This is better appreciated several hours later in the *lower panel,* when contractions, now recorded with a direct catheter, are more regular and doubtless of stronger amplitude. From 8M onward the baseline suggests subtle undulations, perhaps sinusoidal, but there is also the suggestion of an acceleration with manipulation or movement just before 15M and clearly an increase in apparent variability after 29M. This patient had received both narcotics and barbiturates during labor.

Despite the variability, the absence of diminished decelerations during labor precludes the diagnosis of acute fetal asphyxia. In addition, the absence of variable decelerations with overshoot or an unstable baseline are persuasive arguments against any deterioration in the condition of the fetus. Consider medication to the mother, anomaly, or other factors (see tracing 76).

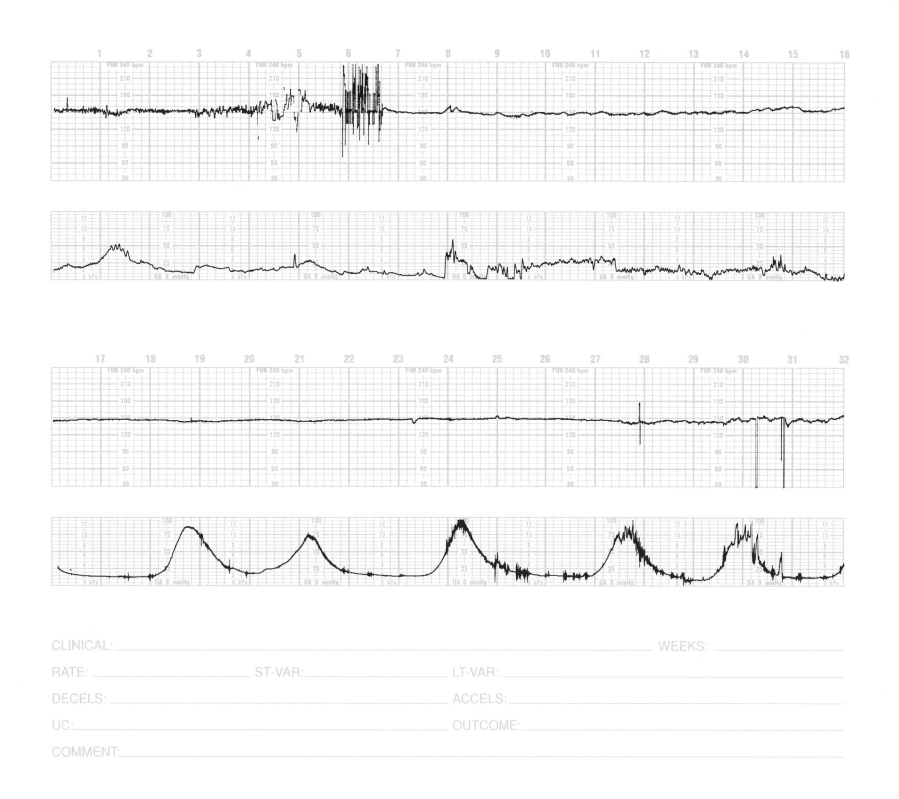

CLINICAL: _____ WEEKS: _____

RATE: _____ ST-VAR: _____ LT-VAR: _____

DECELS: _____ ACCELS: _____

UC: _____ OUTCOME: _____

COMMENT: _____

TRACING: 20

CLINICAL: Maternal fever.

WEEKS: 41

BASELINE RATE: 190–210

STV: Diminished.

LTV: Diminished.

DECELERATIONS: Mild variable.

ACCELERATIONS: Variable ("shoulders").

UC: Second stage.

OUTCOME: Apgar scores, 6/8; normal neonatal course.

COMMENT: This tracing demonstrates baseline tachycardia and modestly decreased short-term variability in an otherwise resilient fetus. Under normal circumstances, when the baseline heart rate rises, both long- and short-term variability diminish. Notice the accelerations that tend to follow the trivial variable decelerations. It is not appropriate to refer to these changes as "overshoot" because of the presence of at least modest amounts of variability, and the erratic, benign-appearing decelerations. True variable decelerations with overshoot demonstrate persistently absent variability and smooth decelerations. Even with maternal fever from chorioamnionitis, most infants are not infected. Fetal monitor patterns may not be reliable signs of early fetal infection and approaches to treatment of fetal tachycardia vary. Despite the maternal fever, the tracing suggests a resilient infant. The newborn should be evaluated for sepsis.

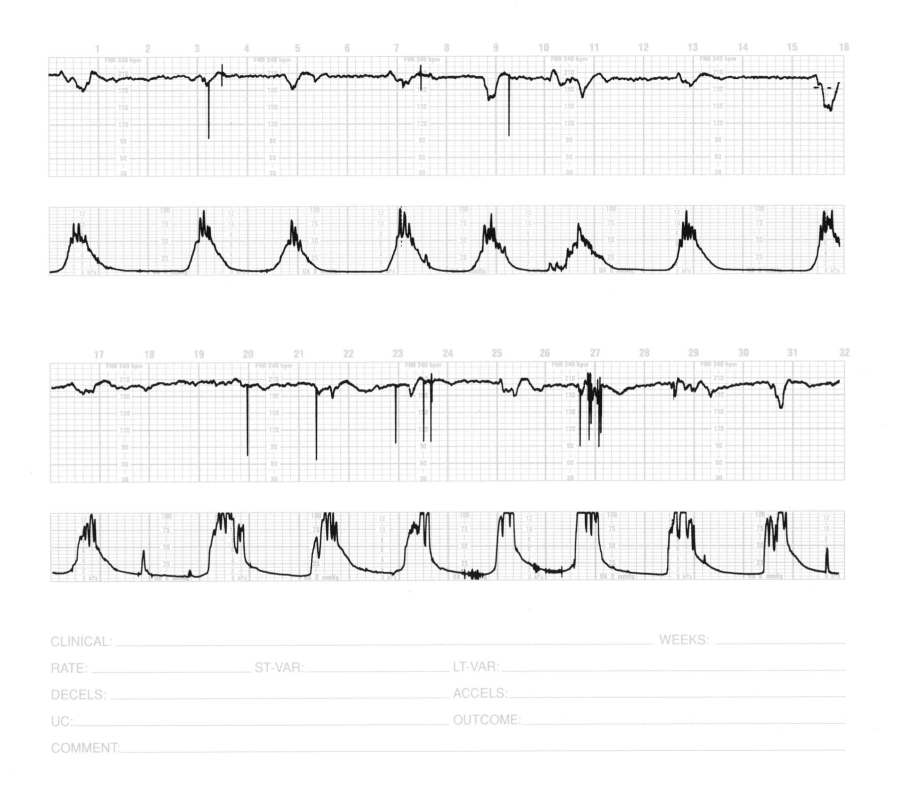

CLINICAL: _____ WEEKS: _____

RATE: _____ ST-VAR: _____ LT-VAR: _____

DECELS: _____ ACCELS: _____

UC: _____ OUTCOME: _____

COMMENT: _____

TRACING: 21

CLINICAL: Hypertension, possibly abruptio placentae.

WEEKS: 34

BASELINE RATE: 170–190.

STV: Decreased.

LTV: Average.

DECELERATIONS: Late (11M–16M).

ACCELERATIONS: Uniform.

UC: Very frequent (possibly oxytocin, possibly abruption).

OUTCOME: Apgar scores, 6/8.

COMMENT: This tracing is unusual in that the external ultrasound transducer was able to trace the FHR at a rate greater than 180 bpm. Frequently, external devices will half-count such high rates. Note the frequent uterine contractions suggestive of abruption. Late decelerations, absent at the beginning of the tracing, appear along with considerable artifact after 10M. Following these late decelerations, the baseline heart rate rises, variability decreases, and the decelerations disappear despite the persistence of the frequent contractions. Does the change in the mother's position from supine to lateral at 22M cause a prolonged fetal deceleration? Or is the fetal heart rate being half-counted? Or is it the mother's heart rate that is being counted? Guess the latter!

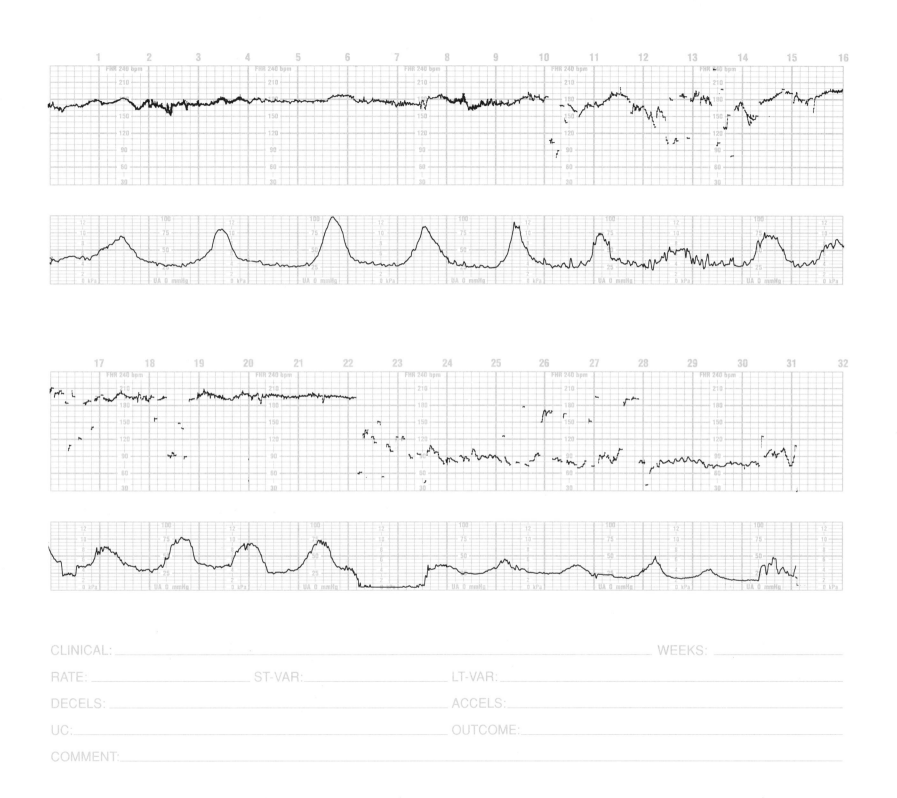

TRACING: 22

CLINICAL: Normal pregnancy, maternal anxiety.

WEEKS: Term.

BASELINE RATE: Hard to determine.

STV: Decreased.

LTV: Decreased.

DECELERATIONS: Small variable.

ACCELERATIONS: Overshoot.

UC: Early labor.

OUTCOME: Normal, IUGR.

COMMENT: This previously normal tracing reveals a rapid rise in heart rate (>50 bpm) over about 8 minutes, unaccompanied by decelerations. Few factors can change the rate this dramatically, and asphyxia is not one of them. This rapid a rise is unlikely to be the result of maternal fever (excluding chills) or beta-mimetic drugs, which elevate the rate much more leisurely. Profound asphyxia would induce bradycardia, not tachycardia. Lesser degrees of asphyxia during labor would produce more obvious late decelerations and eventually a modest elevation in rate—rarely as dramatic as this. Atropine and cholinergic blockade could cause this rapid rate change, but they rarely induce tachycardia above 155 to 170 bpm. Arrhythmia in the form of paroxysmal tachycardia tends to develop far more rapidly, usually over several heartbeats.

In this case, the mother had been given a narcotic (meperidine) and became dysphoric, anxious, and then vomited. The FHR changes seen here developed immediately thereafter. How best to explain this tracing? For want of better explanation, this is "fetal anxiety." Notice that the entire episode lasts about 30 minutes. Although an effect of naloxone (Narcan) cannot be excluded, this sequence of events has been seen without the addition of the narcotic antagonist.

During the tachycardia the variability is markedly diminished with small accelerations and decelerations suggesting overshoot—related to the diminution in parasympathetic tone. The pattern subsides in 20 to 30 minutes. If narcotics have not induced the pattern, they are frequently *effective* in bringing the rate down. This is *not* an asphyxial episode. Notice the exaggerated maternal breathing pattern during contractions after the narcotic has been neutralized.

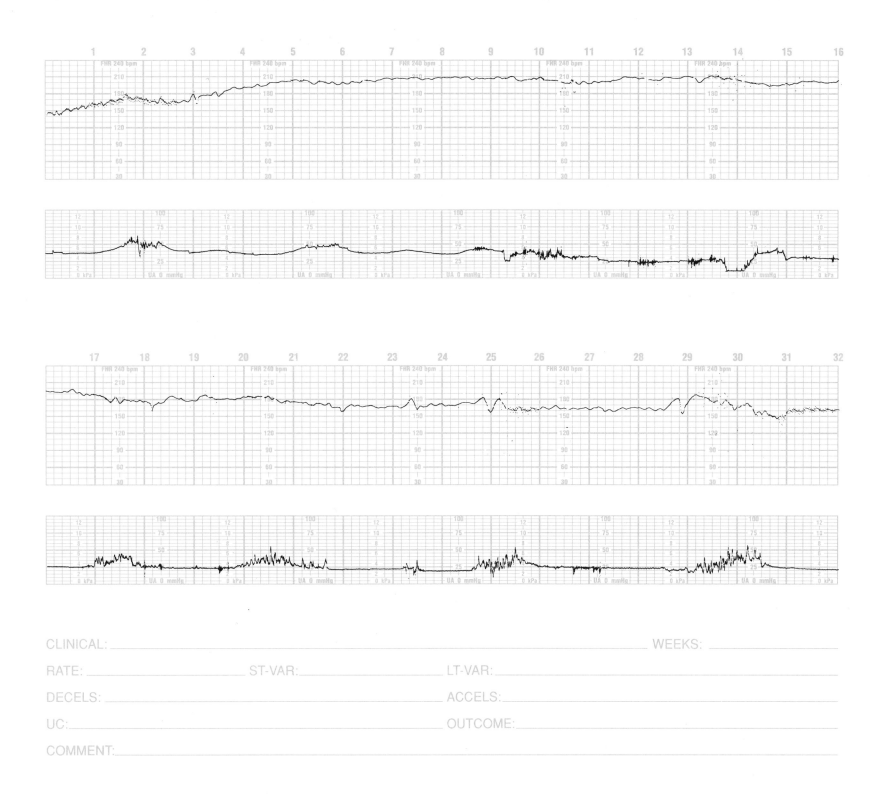

CLINICAL: _____ WEEKS: _____

RATE: _____ ST-VAR: _____ LT-VAR: _____

DECELS: _____ ACCELS: _____

UC: _____ OUTCOME: _____

COMMENT: _____

TRACING: 23

CLINICAL: Severe hypertension, on $MgSO_4$.

WEEKS: 37

BASELINE RATE: 150

STV: Absent.

LTV: Decreased.

DECELERATIONS: Small variables, others possibly late.

ACCELERATIONS: Overshoot.

UC: Late labor, irregular.

OUTCOME: Apgar scores, 4/6, neurologic handicap.

COMMENT: While the changes in the UC channel more readily draw our attention, the FHR tracing is conspicuously abnormal. The abrupt changes in the UC channel at 13M and 20M are related to repositioning of the patient for the fetal scalp sample obtained at 10M. The normal pH of 7.26 gives a clue to the mechanism of the abnormality but belies the tracing's fundamental abnormality. The tracing is marked by absent variability, small variable decelerations with overshoot at 2M, 5M, 13M, and 14M, and the suggestion of late decelerations at 8M, 18M, and 26M. Note the absence of any significant change in the FHR pattern associated with the manipulation of scalp sampling. The somewhat unstable baseline rate in the absence of significant or recurrent decelerations suggests a chronic abnormality (or anomaly) but no acute asphyxial problem as confirmed by the normal pH. The changes seen here are not due to magnesium sulfate. This drug has no consistent effect on heart rate or variability.

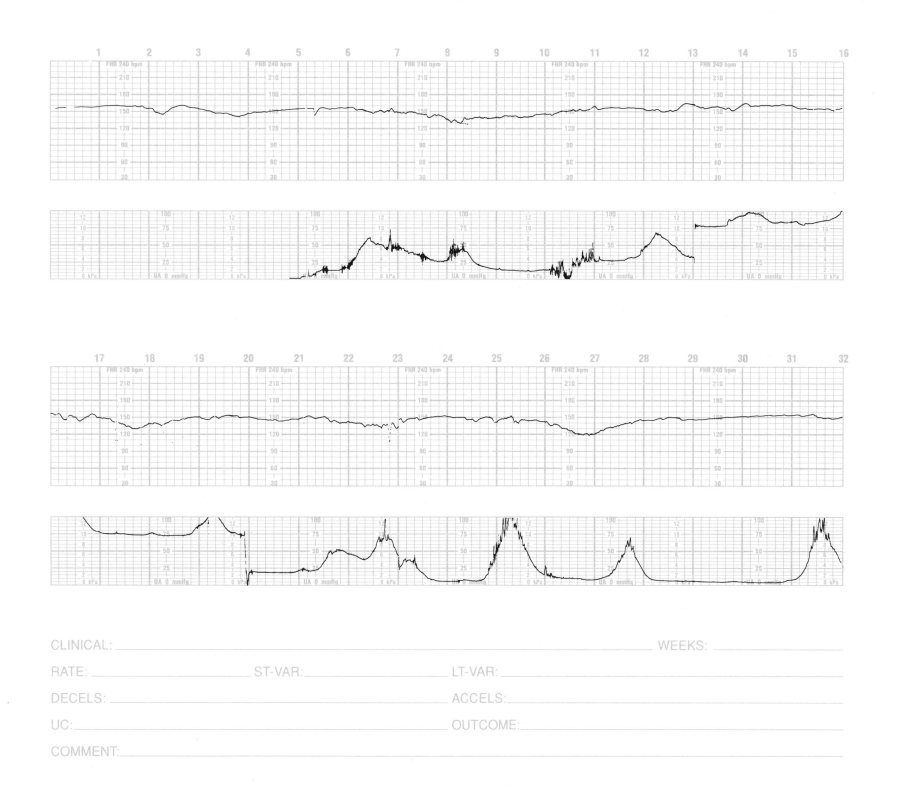

CLINICAL:_____ WEEKS:_____

RATE:_____ ST-VAR:_____ LT-VAR:_____

DECELS:_____ ACCELS:_____

UC:_____ OUTCOME:_____

COMMENT:_____

TRACING: 24

CLINICAL: Positive contraction stress test.

WEEKS: 36

BASELINE RATE: 140

STV: Decreased.

LTV: Decreased.

DECELERATIONS: Late.

ACCELERATIONS: None.

UC: Hypertonus *(upper panel)*—effect of oxytocin, none in lower panel.

OUTCOME: Meconium staining, low Apgar scores, IUGR.

COMMENT: In the *upper tracing,* decelerations appear in response to frequent, poorly recorded, uterine contractions induced by oxytocin. When the oxytocin is removed the contractions and the decelerations disappear. Nevertheless, accelerations do not appear, and the recovery is far from reassuring. During antepartum testing this would be classified as a nonreactive NST, positive CST.

This tracing reveals absent variability. The excursions that mimic variability in this external tracing are all artifact. In general, external transducers exaggerate the amount of variability—they do not reduce it. Therefore, if the tracing appears flat, as in this case, it is likely that the direct electrode will be even flatter. The exaggerated variability around 5M is related to the pelvic examination and the manipulations with the tocotransducer. Irrespective of the estimation of variability, there can be little doubt that accelerations are absent. This is a most troublesome tracing that requires consideration of termination of pregnancy.

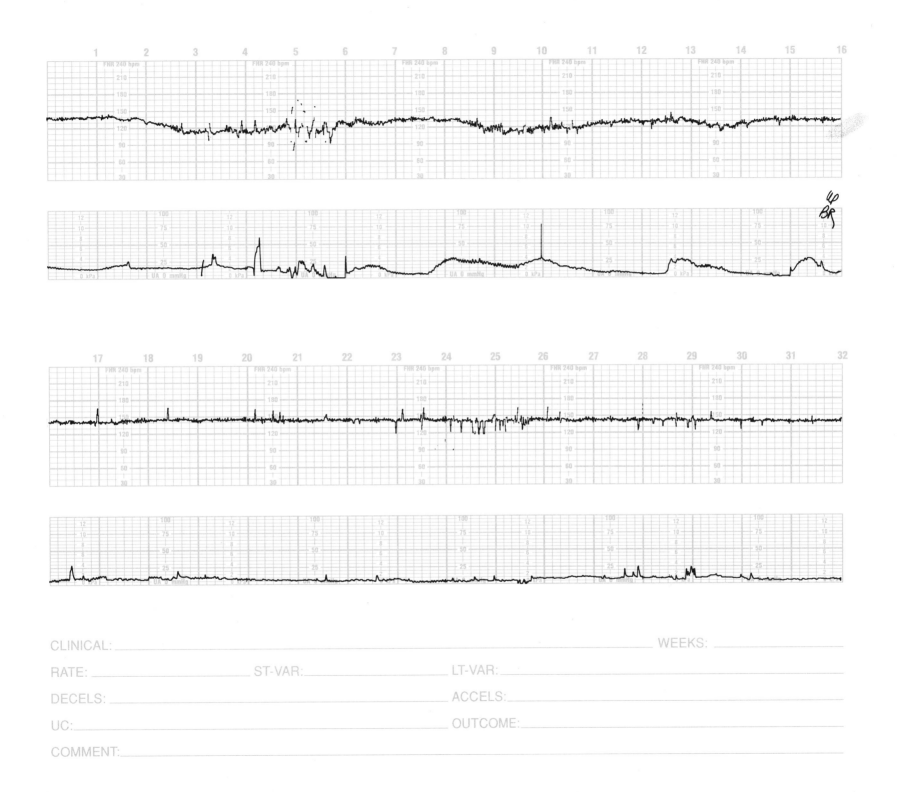

TRACING: 25

CLINICAL: Uneventful prenatal course.

WEEKS: 39

BASELINE RATE: 150

STV: Average.

LTV: Average.

DECELERATIONS: Late.

ACCELERATIONS: None.

UC: Regular, effect of epidural.

OUTCOME: Apgar scores, 9/9; uneventful neonatal course.

COMMENT: This tracing illustrates the development of late decelerations following epidural anesthesia and maternal hypotension. In this previously reassuring tracing, one can easily follow the evolution and resolution of the late decelerations. It is often difficult, however, even in retrospect, to decide on the first late deceleration in a series. Is the deviation at 5M a late deceleration? Often, not-so-definitive late decelerations become recognizable only when subsequent, more characteristic features appear. Notice the increased frequency of contractions immediately after the epidural. During recovery, there is a rise in the baseline and a diminution in the baseline variability along with some decrease in the frequency of contractions. The decelerations should be managed by the administration of oxygen, lateral positioning, hydration, and diminution of oxytocin infusion. At the same time, it is reasonable to presume that in this previously normal fetus, these maneuvers will indeed correct the transient, doubtless inconsequential, episode of distress. Prehydration and the patient's maintenance of a lateral position after the anesthesia will dramatically reduce the incidence of late decelerations.

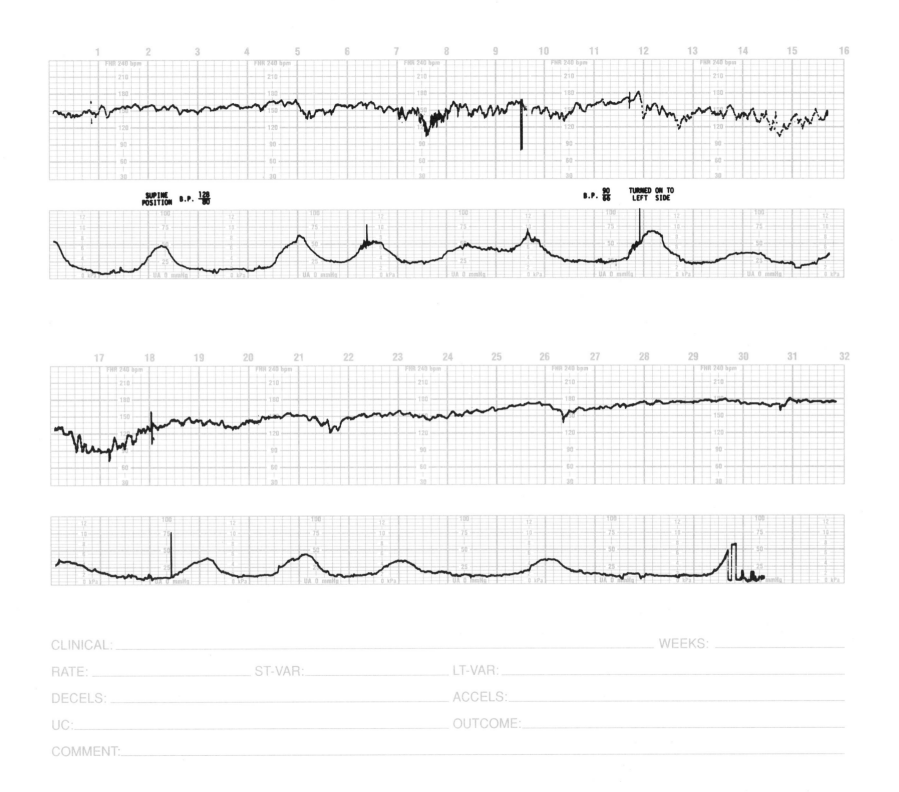

SUPINE
POSITION B.P. 120/80

B.P. 90/65   TURNED ON TO
LEFT SIDE

CLINICAL: _____ WEEKS: _____

RATE: _____ ST-VAR: _____ LT-VAR: _____

DECELS: _____ ACCELS: _____

UC: _____ OUTCOME: _____

COMMENT: _____

TRACING: 26

CLINICAL: Normal pregnancy.

WEEKS: 38

BASELINE RATE: 170–180

STV: Average.

LTV: Average.

DECELERATIONS: Recurrent variable, late.

ACCELERATIONS: None.

UC: Late labor, coupling of contractions, oxytocin effect.

OUTCOME: Emergency cesarean section, Apgar scores, 7/9.

COMMENT: In this previously normal tracing, oxytocin produces excessive uterine contractions. Initially, we see a number of decelerations that suggest late, or more probably variable, decelerations. After 15 minutes, the decelerations become smoother and the variability diminishes, as the baseline returns to its previous level. The latter features exemplify late decelerations. This pattern is temporarily interrupted by the variable deceleration at 22M that swamps the late deceleration. Late decelerations reappear at 23M and 25M. After 26M with the patient on her side, contractions diminishing, and oxygen being administered, the decelerations disappear as the baseline returns to what it was before the episode started. This represents a transient episode of fetal hypoxia with recovery. There is no evidence that such short-lived episodes result in subsequent handicap.

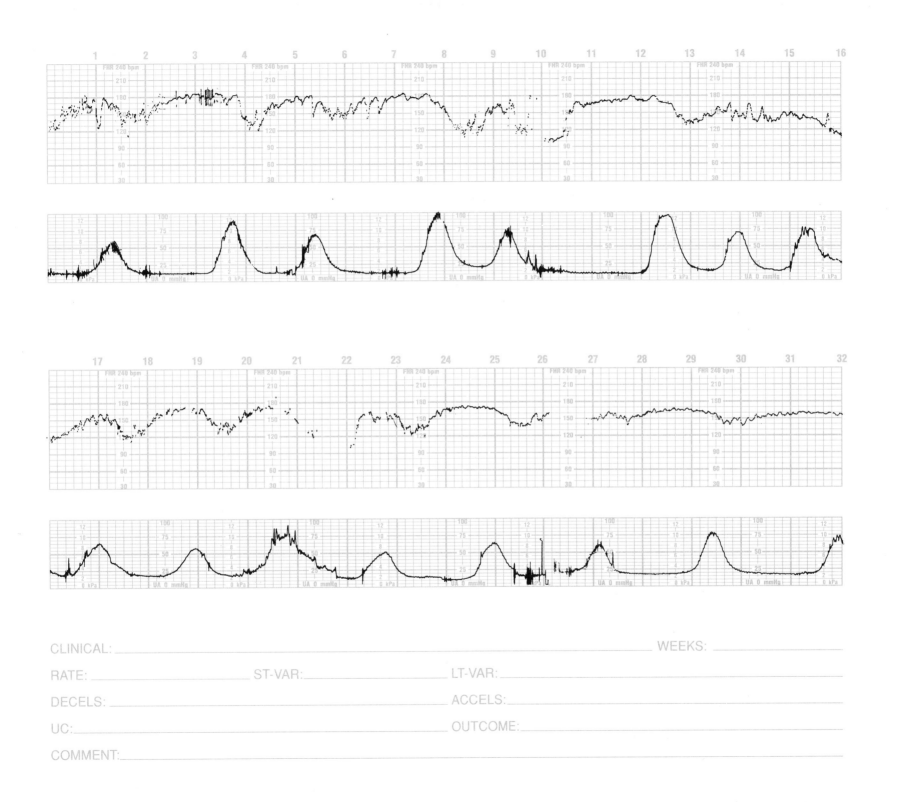

CLINICAL: _____ WEEKS: _____

RATE: _____ ST-VAR: _____ LT-VAR: _____

DECELS: _____ ACCELS: _____

UC: _____ OUTCOME: _____

COMMENT: _____

TRACING: 27

CLINICAL: Late labor—epidural.

WEEKS: 37

BASELINE RATE: 180–190

STV: Decreased, average.

LTV: Decreased, average.

DECELERATIONS: Possibly late, variable.

ACCELERATIONS: None.

UC: Late labor, oxytocin effect.

OUTCOME: Normal Apgar scores.

COMMENT: While there is great temptation to call the decelerations in the *upper panel* late decelerations, careful analysis will reveal considerable variation in (1) the duration of the deceleration and (2) the relationship between the onset of the contractions and the onset of the decelerations. Although there is no tendency for the baseline rate to rise, it is already high and would not likely rise higher even with asphyxia. In the *lower panel* the patient is bearing down. Here we find more obvious decelerations, probably variable, accompanied by an increase in the baseline variability. Notice that the fetal response depends upon the expulsive efforts of the mother. The tachycardia here is unexplained. While each fetus will attempt to maintain a given baseline rate throughout labor, such factors as fever, prolonged labor with inadequate hydration, and maternal anxiety may all conspire to elevate the heart rate of both mother and fetus. The ability of the fetus to maintain or increase short-term variability in the face of decelerations bespeaks a still resilient fetus.

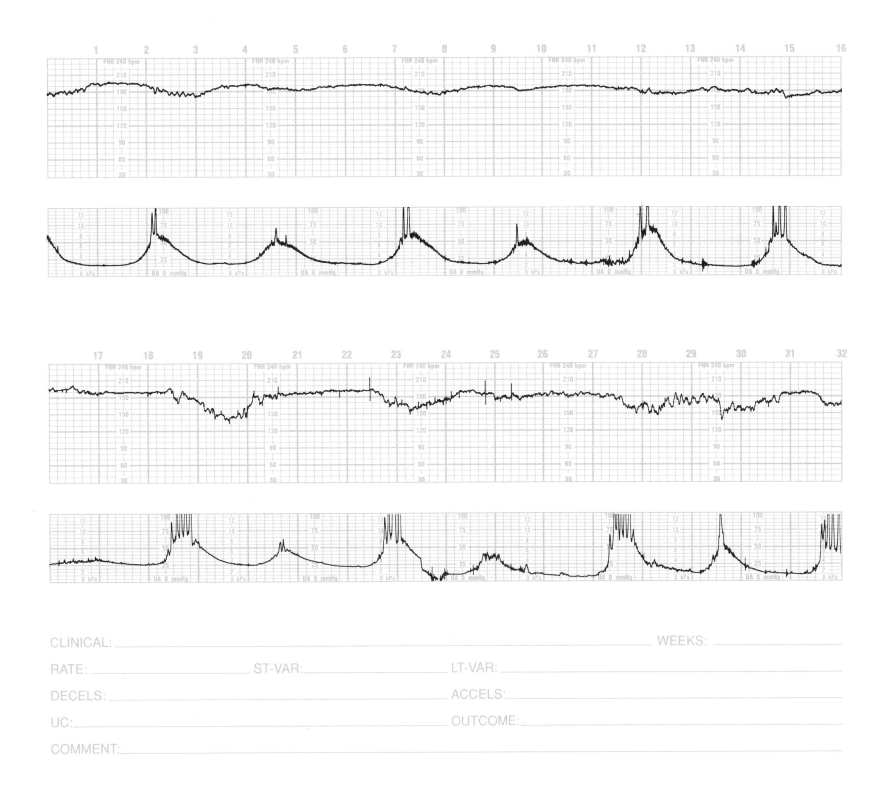

CLINICAL: _____   WEEKS: _____

RATE: _____   ST-VAR: _____   LT-VAR: _____

DECELS: _____   ACCELS: _____

UC: _____   OUTCOME: _____

COMMENT: _____

TRACING: 28

CLINICAL: Normal pregnancy.

WEEKS: 40

BASELINE RATE: 170

STV: Decreased, increased.

LTV: Decreased, average, increased.

DECELERATIONS: Variable.

ACCELERATIONS: Sporadic.

UC: Late labor—oxytocin effect.

OUTCOME: Normal.

COMMENT: While the initial (possibly late) deceleration and decreased variability imply asphyxial distress, these findings are not continued. The first deceleration represents either an isolated variable deceleration or the last of a series of late decelerations. The initial deceleration does not repeat and there is even a short acceleration with undershoot (lambda pattern) at 7M. The initial deceleration is either related to pushing or an examination and should be classified as a variable deceleration. The decreased variability at this time is due to narcotic effect. Thus, the remainder of the *upper panel* can only represent a stable condition or complete recovery.

The *lower panel* is obtained shortly after the *upper panel.* Although the frequency of contractions does not change between *upper* and *lower panels,* the amount of expulsive effort increases considerably. This activity in the second stage increases both the variability and the frequency of decelerations. The decelerations usually develop late in the contraction cycle but differ markedly from each other in duration and proportionality to the underlying uterine contraction.

Notice the absence of a deceleration at 17M. The coupling of the first two contractions plus the expulsive efforts probably contribute to the deceleration at 19M. When the expulsive efforts are diminished (27M), the deceleration becomes considerably smaller. Notice the minimal impact of the vomiting at 28M on the FHR pattern, but the immediate reappearance of a deceleration with the subsequent contraction. The responsiveness of the fetus to these expulsive efforts (premature as they are) and the absence of a rising baseline or decreasing variability preclude significant compromise or deterioration. Expediting the delivery is unnecessary with such patterns.

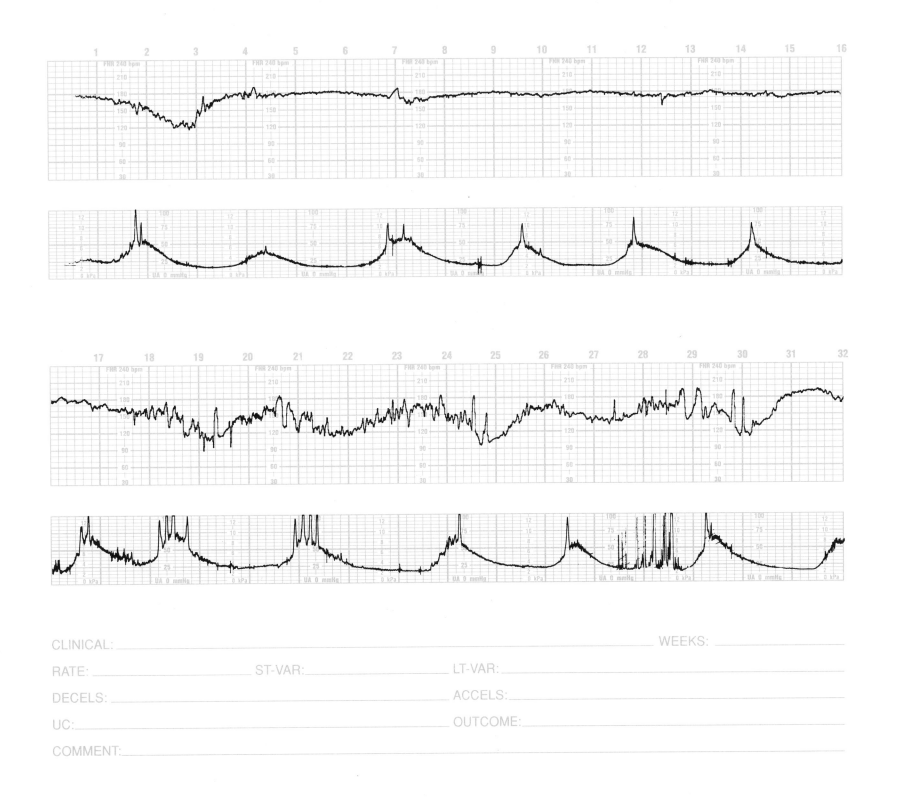

TRACING: 29

CLINICAL: Uneventful prenatal course.

WEEKS: 40

BASELINE RATE: 170–180

STV: Average.

LTV: Average.

DECELERATIONS: Variable or late?

ACCELERATIONS: None.

UC: Second stage.

OUTCOME: Apgar scores, 7/9; occiput anterior to nuchal cord; uneventful neonatal course.

COMMENT: This tracing tests the definition of late decelerations, especially in the second stage. In this situation recurrent decelerations are associated with virtually every contraction. The less dramatic the pushing, however, the less obvious is the deceleration. Indeed, the decelerations disappear entirely when the bearing-down efforts of the mother cease (27M). Similarly, with this frequency of late decelerations, we would expect a rising baseline and loss of variability, neither of which prevail here. While the baseline is already elevated, the variability remains reassuring. Whether this pattern indeed represents variable decelerations from cord compression, mimicking late decelerations, or whether this pattern reflects mild fetal hypoxemia associated with bearing-down efforts and nuchal cord remains to be elucidated. As a minimum the stability of the baseline rate and the maintenance of variability suggest a well-compensated fetus, if indeed there was any significant stress at all. Discontinuation of pushing resolves the problem.

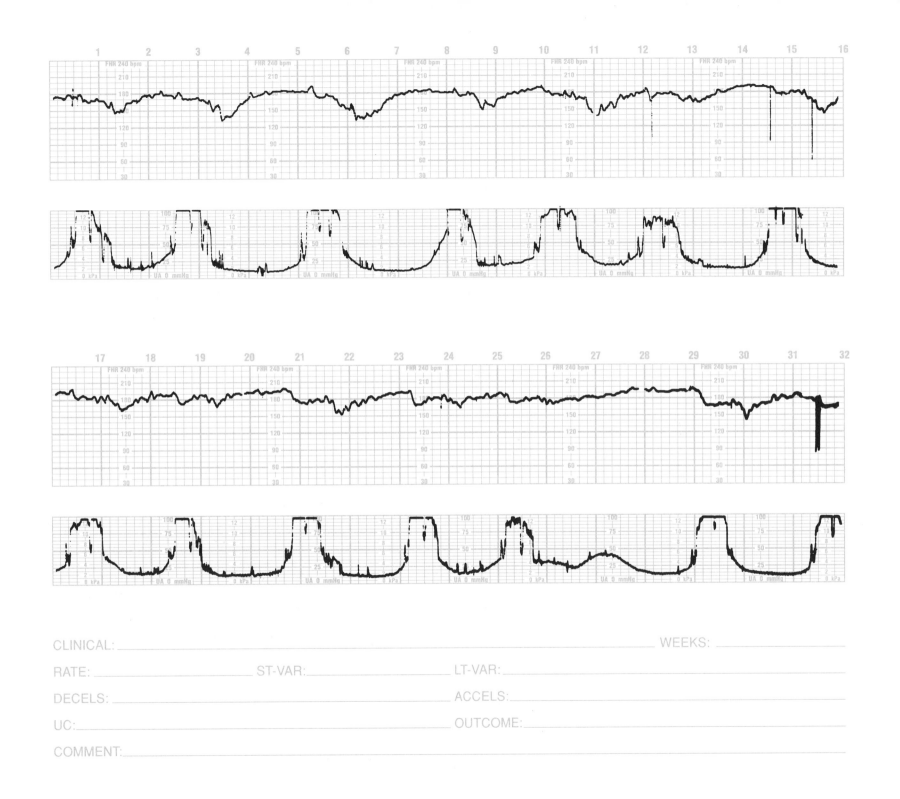

CLINICAL: _____ WEEKS: _____

RATE: _____ ST-VAR:_____ LT-VAR:_____

DECELS: _____ ACCELS:_____

UC:_____ OUTCOME:_____

COMMENT:_____

TRACING: 30

CLINICAL: Both: uneventful prenatal course.

WEEKS: Both: 38

BASELINE RATE: A: 170–180. B: 150

STV: A: Decreased. B: Average.

LTV: A: Decreased. B: Average.

DECELERATIONS: A: Late. B: Prolonged.

ACCELERATIONS: Both: absent.

UC: A: Irregular, early labor. B: Tachysystole, effect of epidural.

OUTCOME: Both: normal Apgar scores, uneventful neonatal course.

COMMENT: Panels A and B represent different fetuses. In the *upper panel,* epidural was administered 20 minutes earlier. Notice the recurrent late decelerations with the larger contractions and the far less obvious decelerations associated with the smaller contractions. Variability is diminished and the baseline rate elevated as a compensatory response to the transient, mild hypoxemia induced by maternal hypotension. The pattern ultimately responds to hydration, turning the patient on her left side, and administration of oxygen. In the majority of instances, such changes can be prevented by preliminary hydration and avoidance of the supine position.

In the *lower panel,* the previously administered alphaprodine (Nisentil) induced a characteristic sinusoidal heart rate pattern. An epidural block, administered 6 minutes previously, characteristically induced an episode of uterine hypertonus. About half the time hypertonus will induce periods of transient, fetal decelerations. These decelerations may appear as characteristic late decelerations or somewhat more prolonged or coupled decelerations. The interval between contractions increases following the episode of hypertonus. The absence of further decelerations and the minimal reactive tachycardia after the deceleration suggest that this brief episode did not adversely impact on this fetus.

78

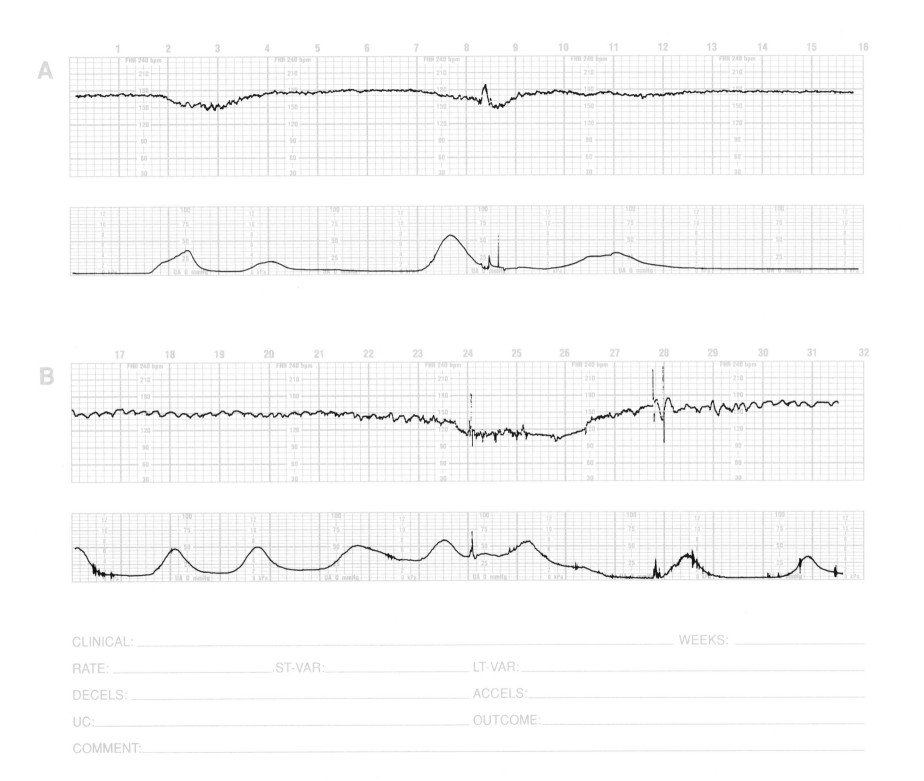

TRACING: 31

CLINICAL: Uneventful pregnancy.

WEEKS: 41

BASELINE RATE: 130–140

STV: Average.

LTV: Average.

DECELERATIONS: Prolonged, late.

ACCELERATIONS: Sporadic, variable ("shoulders").

UC: Hypertonus, tachysystole.

OUTCOME: Apgar scores, 7/8; normal neonatal course.

COMMENT: This tracing illustrates the typical appearance of paracervical block bradycardia. The *top panel* reveals the uterus contracting frequently. Considerable artifact punctuates the FHR channel, probably related to manipulation and examination, but throughout, the fetus maintains a stable baseline rate and variability. The end of the panel reveals variable decelerations. Following the administration of the paracervical block at 17M we see simultaneous uterine hypertonus and a profound deceleration to 60 bpm, which requires about 8 minutes to recover. Notice the spacing out of the contractions and the appearance of late decelerations during recovery. By 32M the FHR pattern is recovering to an expectedly higher rate and decreased variability. Thirty minutes later, it will return to its previous rate and variability.

It is axiomatic, in obstetrical care, that potentially compromising techniques, such as oxytocin stimulation, or paracervical block, be restricted to use in the demonstrably normal fetus. If one were not aware of the preceding reassuring pattern when confronting the pattern at 20M, there would be no basis for intervention or expectancy. The preceding normal FHR pattern warrants the conservative approach as long as the insult (the uterine hypertonus) can be eliminated and the fetus manifests recovery.

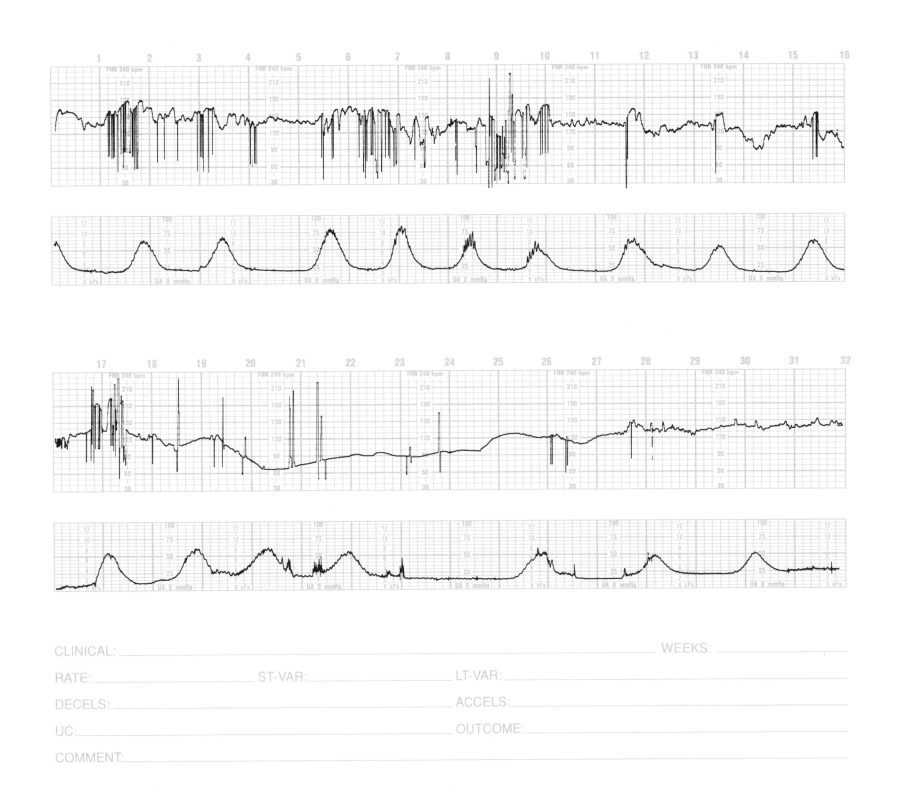

CLINICAL: _____   WEEKS: _____

RATE: _____   ST-VAR: _____   LT-VAR: _____

DECELS: _____   ACCELS: _____

UC: _____   OUTCOME: _____

COMMENT: _____

TRACING: 32

CLINICAL: Uneventful prenatal course.

WEEKS: 38

BASELINE RATE: 135

STV: Decreased.

LTV: Average.

DECELERATIONS: Prolonged, with arrhythmia.

ACCELERATIONS: None.

UC: Early labor.

OUTCOME: Apgar scores, 9/9; uneventful neonatal course.

COMMENT: This tracing illustrates an unusual fetal response to paracervical block anesthesia. Most prolonged decelerations associated with paracervical block are accompanied by uterine hypertonus but unassociated with arrhythmia. These limited, beat-to-beat arrhythmias suggest a response to catecholamines. Identical patterns may be seen in either mother or fetus following administration of beta-mimetic tocolytics or local anesthetics via other routes (i.e., intravenously, epidural). The episodes are usually quite short-lived, returning promptly to the previous heart rate pattern. No further investigation is warranted and deterioration with this pattern is essentially unheard of.

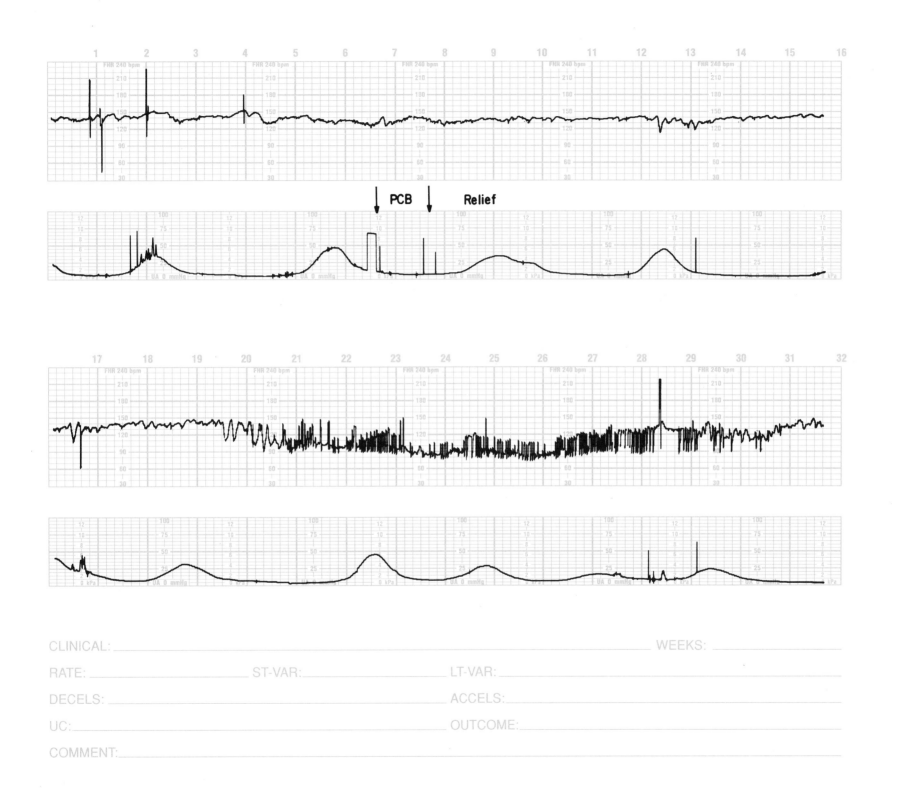

PCB   Relief

TRACING: 33

CLINICAL: Both: uneventful.

WEEKS: A: 38. B: 40.

BASELINE RATE: A: 140. B: 150.

STV: Both: average.

LTV: Both: average.

DECELERATIONS: Both: prolonged, late.

ACCELERATIONS: Both: none.

UC: A: Hypertonus. B: Tetany.

OUTCOME: Both: Normal Apgar scores, uneventful neonatal course.

COMMENT: These tracings illustrate iatrogenic distress in two fetuses. In the *upper panel,* the combination of epidural anesthesia, supine hypotension, and oxytocin, produces excessive uterine activity and obvious late decelerations. Notice the exaggerated variability associated with late decelerations and the sustained deceleration associated with the prolonged contraction. A late deceleration develops as the heart rate recovers to a higher baseline rate and diminished variability. With prompt curtailment of the oxytocin, adequate hydration, and resumption of the lateral position, the pattern recovers. The duration of the compensatory tachycardia and decreased variability are proportional to the severity of the asphyxial insult.

In the *lower panel,* the deceleration appears almost simultaneously with the tetanic contraction. The rate remains above 60 bpm and variability is maintained. During recovery, late decelerations, reactive tachycardia, and diminished variability appear. (Forty minutes later the pattern returned to normal. Despite the curtailment of oxytocin, frequent uterine contractions persisted for about 20 minutes.) Oxytocin first increases the frequency, not the amplitude, of contractions. If the contractions become too frequent, the resting tone between contractions rises. With further increases in the dosage the amplitude may rise and the contractions coalesce with persistent elevation of tonus. Although the half-life of oxytocin is short—about 3 minutes—the effects of overdosage may last significantly longer and may have damaging effects on the fetus. In the vast majority of cases, however, such transient episodes of asphyxia recover completely and do not compromise outcome.

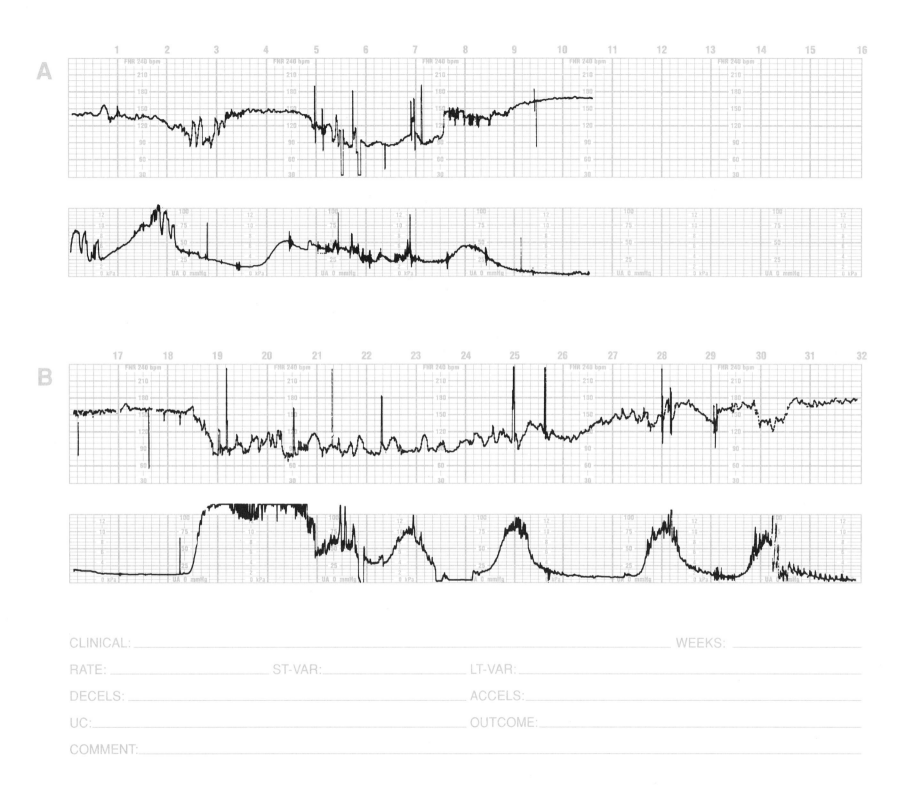

CLINICAL: _____ WEEKS: _____

RATE: _____ ST-VAR: _____ LT-VAR: _____

DECELS: _____ ACCELS: _____

UC: _____ OUTCOME: _____

COMMENT: _____

TRACING: 34

CLINICAL: Uneventful prenatal course.

WEEKS: 41

BASELINE RATE: 130

STV: Average.

LTV: Average.

DECELERATIONS: Prolonged.

ACCELERATIONS: Variable.

UC: Effect of position change.

OUTCOME: Apgar scores, 8/9; uneventful neonatal course.

COMMENT: This tracing illustrates the appearance of isolated, prolonged decelerations that arise without prior warning in a patient in the supine position. The *upper panel* tracing could not be more reassuring. Contractions are frequent but irregular both in amplitude, duration, and interval. Without warning a deceleration appears that lasts for several minutes then returns promptly to the previous baseline, or slightly above, associated with transient diminution in baseline variability. The deceleration prompts turning the patient on her left side and the administration of oxygen. These maneuvers contribute to the amelioration of the pattern as well as the spacing out of uterine contractions.

There is no prevailing consensus on the management of these intermittent, recoverable, prolonged decelerations. One paradigm suggests that they can probably be discounted, providing that the baseline variability and rate return to their previous normal pattern. Another suggests that if such decelerations repeat, intervention must be considered.

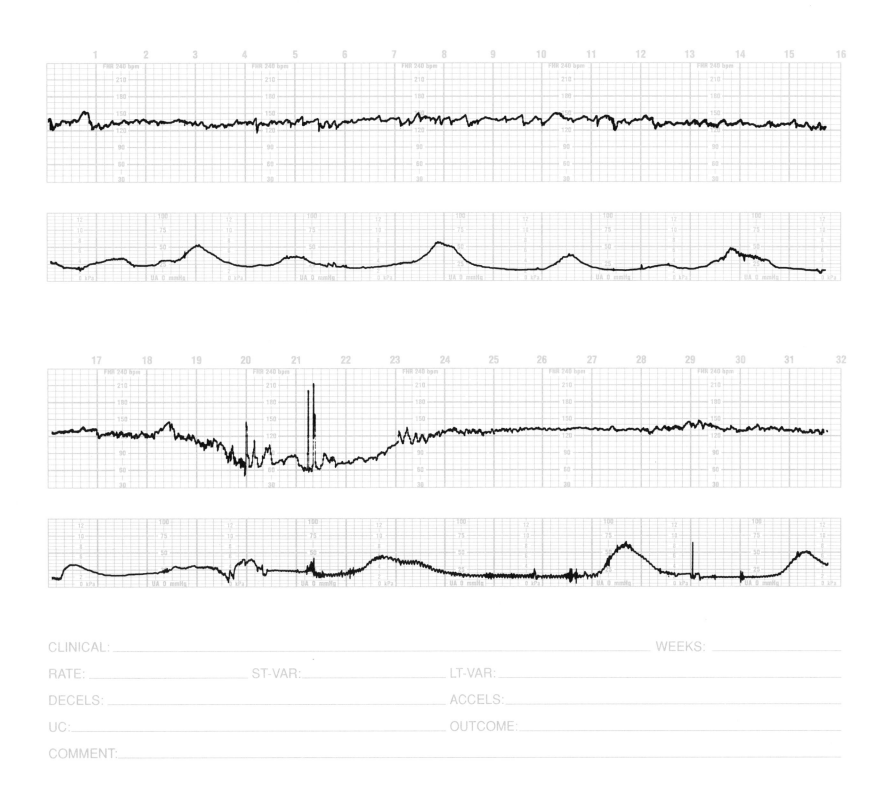

TRACING: 35

CLINICAL: Preeclampsia, dysfunctional labor.

WEEKS: 40

BASELINE RATE: 120–130

STV: Average.

LTV: Average.

DECELERATIONS: Early, variable, prolonged.

ACCELERATIONS: Variable ("shoulders").

UC: Second stage.

OUTCOME: Apgar scores, 9/9; uneventful neonatal course.

COMMENT: This tracing illustrates FHR patterns during the second stage in a primigravida woman whose cervix has been fully dilated for 2 hours, with the fetus in occiput-anterior position. In the *upper panel,* frequent uterine contractions and bearing-down efforts induce early (possibly variable) decelerations. Despite this exertion, the fetus maintains a stable baseline rate and average variability. At 20M, the combination of frequent contractions, compulsive, expulsive efforts, and descent produce marked and dramatic change in the heart rate. Despite this, the fetus maintains abundant variability and dramatic accelerations. Although a number of maneuvers were tried, including repositioning to right and left sides, Trendelenburg position, and the administration of oxygen, none influenced the heart rate pattern. The more appropriate maneuver would have been to have the patient stop pushing. The infant was delivered 30 minutes later.

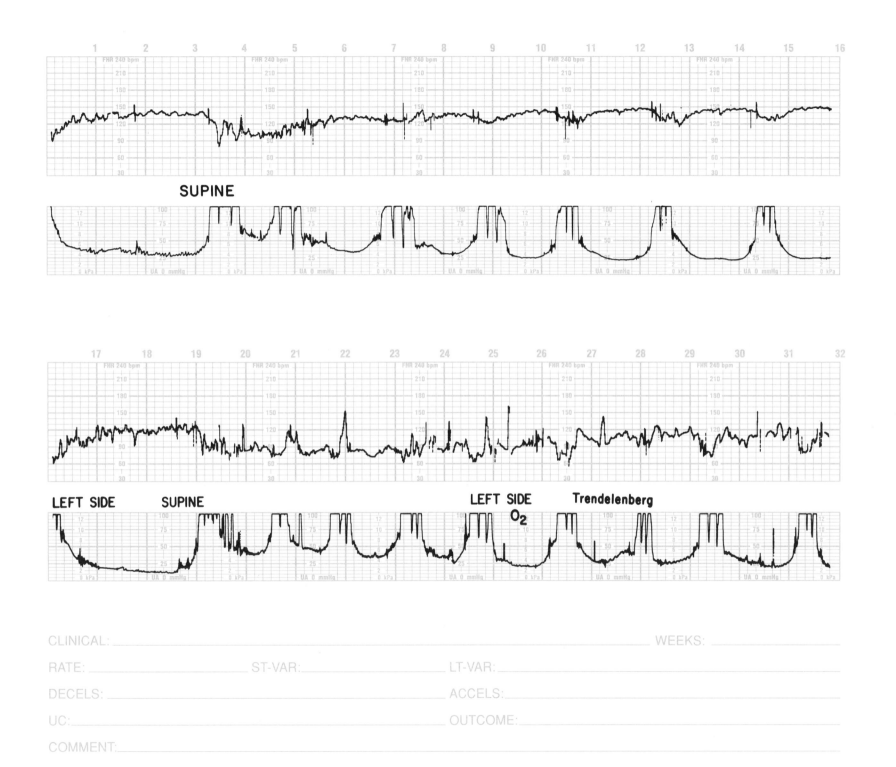

SUPINE

LEFT SIDE   SUPINE   LEFT SIDE   Trendelenberg
O₂

CLINICAL: _____   WEEKS: _____

RATE: _____   ST-VAR: _____   LT-VAR: _____

DECELS: _____   ACCELS: _____

UC: _____   OUTCOME: _____

COMMENT: _____

TRACING: 36

CLINICAL: Normal pregnancy.

WEEKS: 39

BASELINE RATE: 160–170

STV: Average.

LTV: Average.

DECELERATIONS: Variable, prolonged.

ACCELERATIONS: Variable, spontaneous.

UC: Early labor, hypertonus—effect of epidural anesthesia, shivering superimposed on tracing.

OUTCOME: Normal.

COMMENT: This tracing presents some FHR responses to epidural anesthesia. The tracing suggests decelerations at 3M and 12M associated with prolonged contractions. The sustained variability and the stable baseline heart rate from 14M onward suggests no significant compromise if no further assault is added. But additional compromise is manifested in the form of hypotension, shivering, and excessive uterine activity. These findings, including the hypertonus, are common after epidural anesthesia and may induce the dramatic decelerations seen here. They may be modified to a great extent by limited analgesia, prehydration, and lateral uterine displacement. The deceleration at 20M appears shortly after the onset of shivering. After 26M, the diversion of uterine blood flow from the very frequent contractions and the shivering preclude fetal recovery.

Although shivering introduces considerable artifact into the tracing, the details of the deceleration remain clearly discernible. Given the normal tracing prior to administration of the epidural and the resilience of the fetus during the decelerations, the tracing will likely recover with conservative measures. Turning the patient on her side, applying warm blankets, and supporting her blood pressure will likely return the tracing to normal.

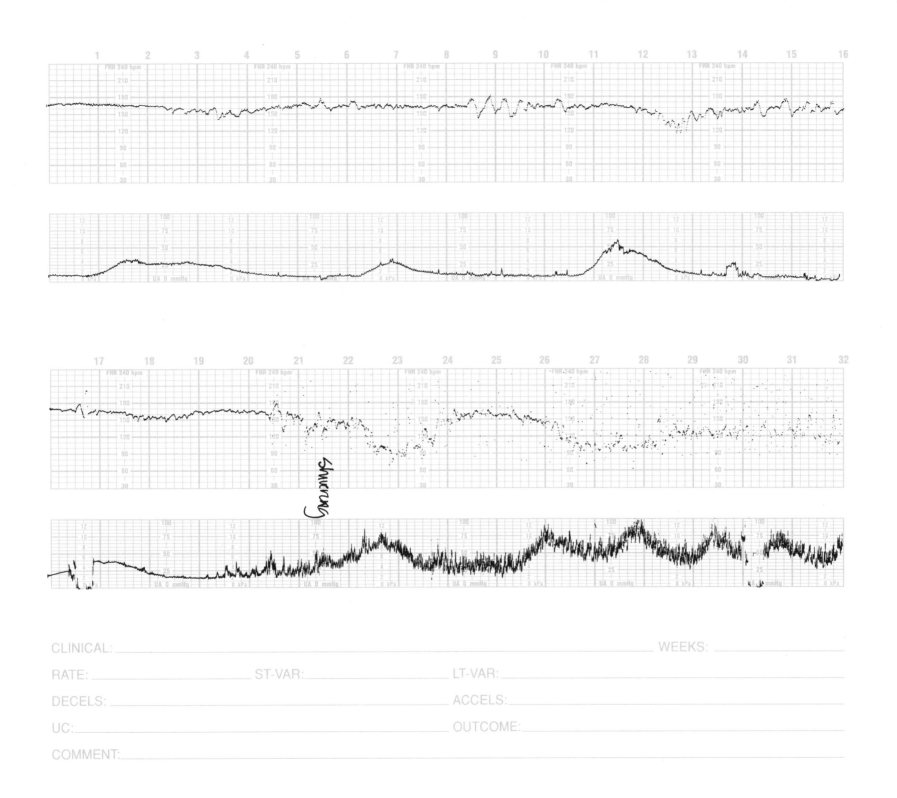

TRACING: 37

CLINICAL: Oligohydramnios, meconium staining.

WEEKS: 38

BASELINE RATE: 125

STV: Average.

LTV: Average.

DECELERATIONS: Prolonged.

ACCELERATIONS: Sporadic.

UC: Irregular, early labor—poorly recorded.

OUTCOME: Meconium staining, dysmature; Apgar scores, 3/8; normal outcome.

COMMENT: This is a typical pattern in a resilient, postmature fetus. Note the small accelerations associated with contractions at 2M, and probably 13M and 19M. Note also the normal baseline rate, increased short-term variability, and broad, shallow decelerations at 4M and 19M. These should be considered prolonged, not late, decelerations. The duration of the decelerations is out of proportion to the duration of the uterine contractions. The contraction at 26M produces no comparable response. The most likely explanation of these prolonged decelerations is either cord compression from the associated oligohydramnios or fetal breathing movements.

Although one has the reasonable expectation of a healthy fetus in this situation, induction of labor with constant fetal surveillance may reasonably be undertaken. If decreased amniotic fluid volume is found, as in this case, consideration may be given to amnioinfusion therapy.

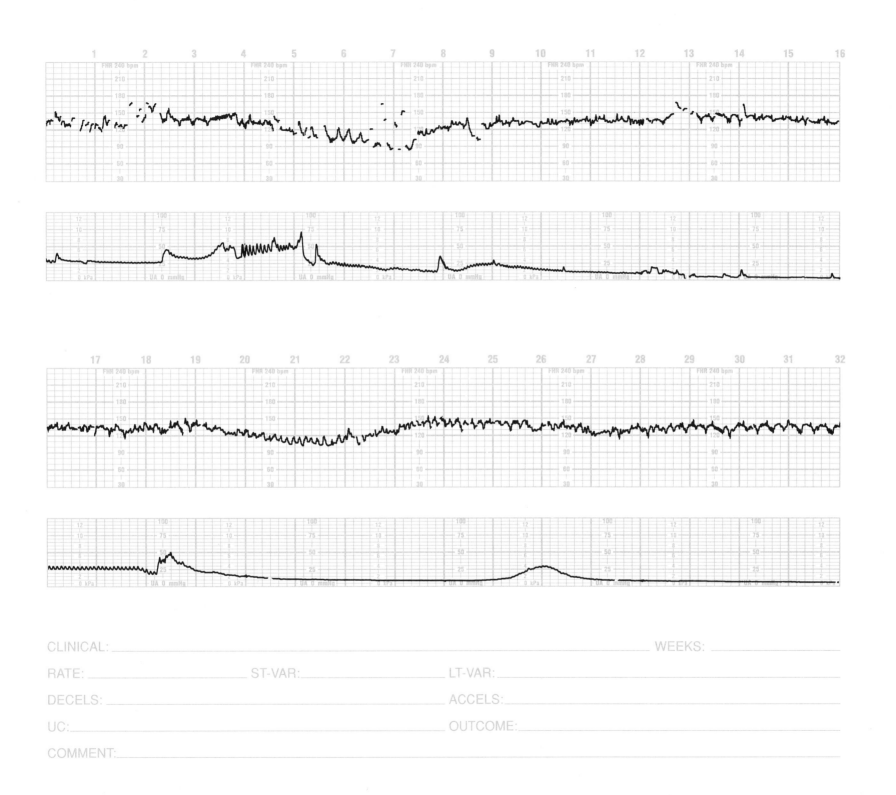

TRACING: 38

CLINICAL: Postdate pregnancy, early labor, oligohydramnios.

WEEKS: 43

BASELINE RATE: 110–120

STV: Average, increased.

LTV: Average.

DECELERATIONS: Prolonged, variable.

ACCELERATIONS: Variable.

UC: Irregular.

OUTCOME: Meconium staining, postmaturity syndrome, normal outcome.

COMMENT: This pattern, obtained in a postdate pregnancy, reveals a low baseline rate, normal to increased variability, and broad, shallow decelerations along with variable decelerations. The decelerations should not be classified as late; they vary considerably in duration, amplitude, and relationship to the underlying contraction. The baseline shows no tendency toward tachycardia. While these features tend to deny a fetal indication for intervention, more decelerations should be expected later in labor. These findings, present during antepartum testing in the term or postdate fetus, are now considered sufficient indication for termination of pregnancy by induction of labor. Compare this tracing with tracing 37.

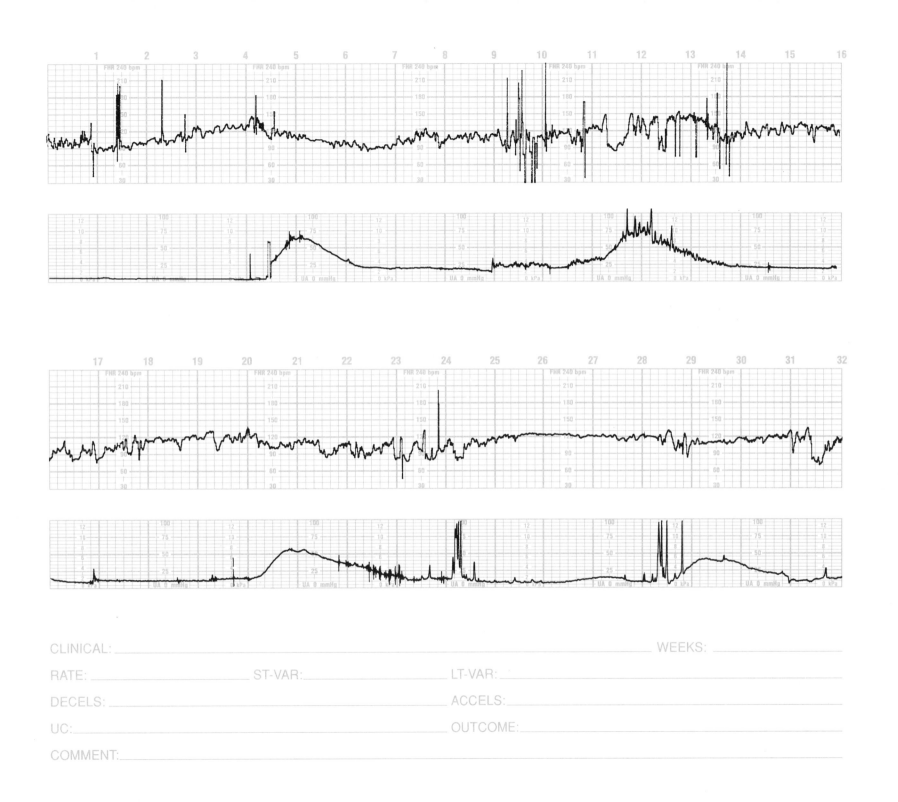

TRACING: 39

CLINICAL: Normal pregnancy.

WEEKS: 40

BASELINE RATE: 150

STV: Average.

LTV: Average, increased.

DECELERATIONS: Variable.

ACCELERATIONS: Variable ("shoulders").

UC: Spontaneous active labor.

OUTCOME: Normal.

COMMENT: This tracing illustrates several features of variable decelerations including their intermittent nature, variable pattern, and coassociation with variable accelerations ("shoulders"). Exaggerated long-term variability (saltatory) pattern is especially likely at the end of the deceleration. Most decelerations are anticipated by a variable acceleration followed by a rather abrupt downslope, occasionally culminating at 20M and 26M in a brief episode of asystole (heart block). Note the dramatic differences between the patterns at the bases of these two variable decelerations (please do not call them "severe"). In the deceleration at 20M, the heart rate stabilizes temporarily above 60 bpm and reveals exaggerated variability (probably some ectopic beats as well). In the deceleration at 26M, the heart rate stabilizes below 60 bpm and reveals the characteristic pattern of nodal rhythm, with its brief deceleration and subtle warmup. In both instances, the return to baseline is erratic but prompt, with rapid recovery of the baseline rate and variability. Thus, the pattern at the base of the deceleration carries little prognostic value but, simply reflects the mechanism of cardiac pacing (nodal or sinus). These changes, in turn, reflect the level to which the rate descends. Thus, the variable deceleration at 26M is not "more severe" or "more ominous" than the deceleration at 20M. Occasionally, as in this patient after 27M, such exaggerated decelerations produce a small drop in the baseline rate but no real diminution in variability. These frequent decelerations early in labor suggest compression of the umbilical cord from occult prolapse, nuchal cord, or membranous insertion of the cord. While the tracing, strictly speaking, does not bespeak fetal deterioration or compromise, the likelihood of these decelerations recurring later on is considerable. This fetus was delivered vaginally; the placenta revealed membranous insertion of the cord.

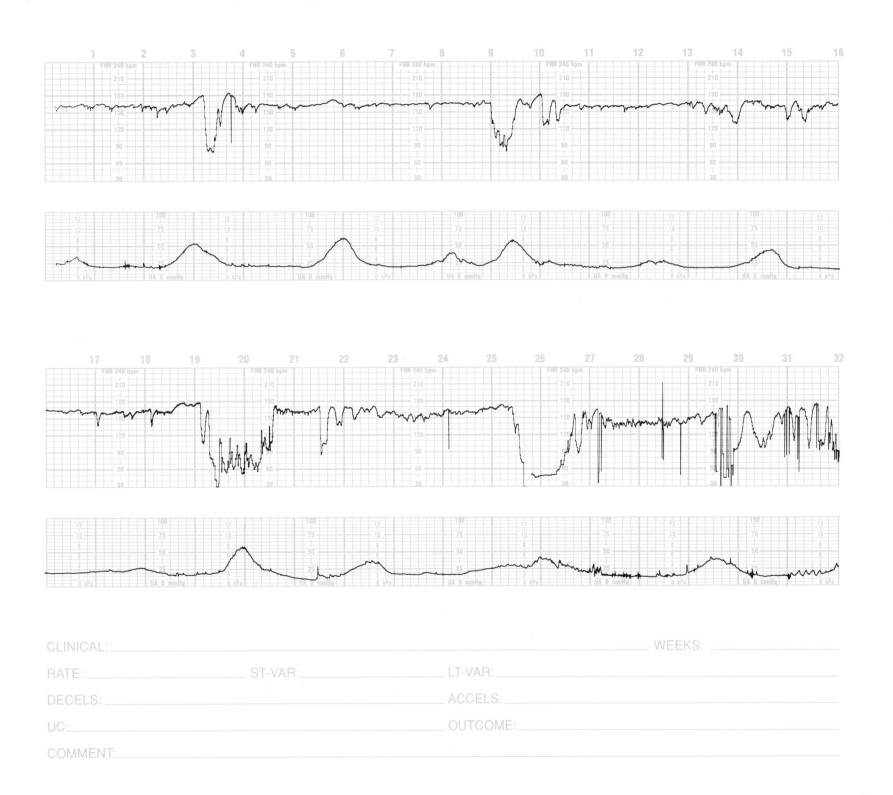

TRACING: 40

CLINICAL: Normal pregnancy.

WEEKS: Term

BASELINE RATE: 145–150

STV: Average.

LTV: Average.

DECELERATIONS: Variable.

ACCELERATIONS: Variable ("shoulders").

UC: Active phase of labor.

OUTCOME: Normal.

COMMENT: This tracing reveals a sinusoidal pattern following the administration of alphaprodine (Nisentil) to the mother. Notice that the oscillations are not perfectly regular. They persist into the beginning of a variable deceleration at 3M and continue thereafter. The amplitude of the oscillations is increased in response to the decelerations and is diminished (damped) thereafter. The variable decelerations are usually preceded by a variable acceleration ("shoulders")—a reassuring sign. Note the increasing patient reaction to the contraction—the activity at peaks of the contractions—as the medication wears off. Sinusoidal patterns associated with narcotic administration to the mother are benign and readily reversed by naloxone (Narcan).

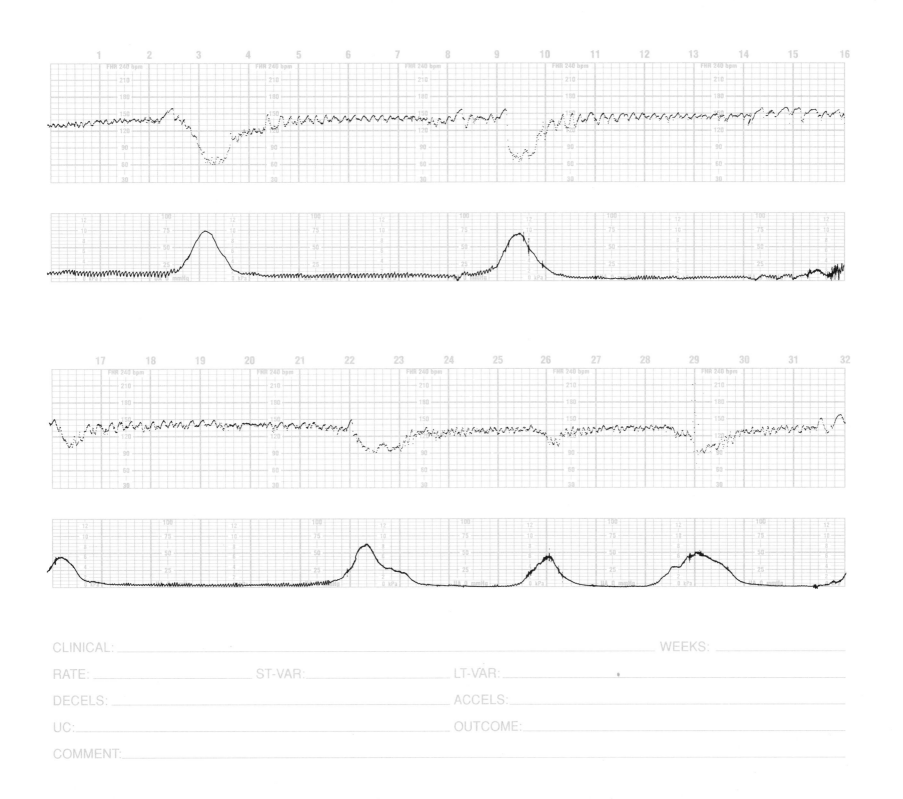

CLINICAL: _____ WEEKS: _____

RATE: _____ ST-VAR: _____ LT-VAR: _____

DECELS: _____ ACCELS: _____

UC: _____ OUTCOME: _____

COMMENT: _____

TRACING: 41

CLINICAL: A: Normal, occiput posterior (OP). B: Normal, occiput anterior (OA).

WEEKS: Both: term

BASELINE RATE: A: 180. B: 170.

STV: Both: average.

LTV: Both: average.

DECELERATIONS: Both: variable.

ACCELERATIONS: Both: variable ("shoulders").

UC: Both: late labor with pushing.

OUTCOME: Both: normal Apgar scores.

COMMENT: These two panels obtained during the second stage of labor in different fetuses reveal second-stage decelerations, which may vary considerably depending upon the position of the fetal head. The occiput posterior position tends to reveal isolated, limited decelerations of considerable amplitude as registered in the *upper panel*. Despite the frequent decelerations, the baseline rate and variability remain stable. Notice the correspondence of the expulsive efforts and the deceleration pattern at 5M, 9M, and 10M. During the second stage, variable decelerations are more likely to represent head compression than cord compression.

In the *lower panel* the fetal head is in the occiput anterior position. Here the decelerations tend to be of lesser amplitude than those in the occiput anterior position, but the decelerations tend to be longer, less well-defined, and sometimes simulate late decelerations as they do at 18M, 21M, and 25M. Neither pattern warrants intervention or modification of the expulsive efforts.

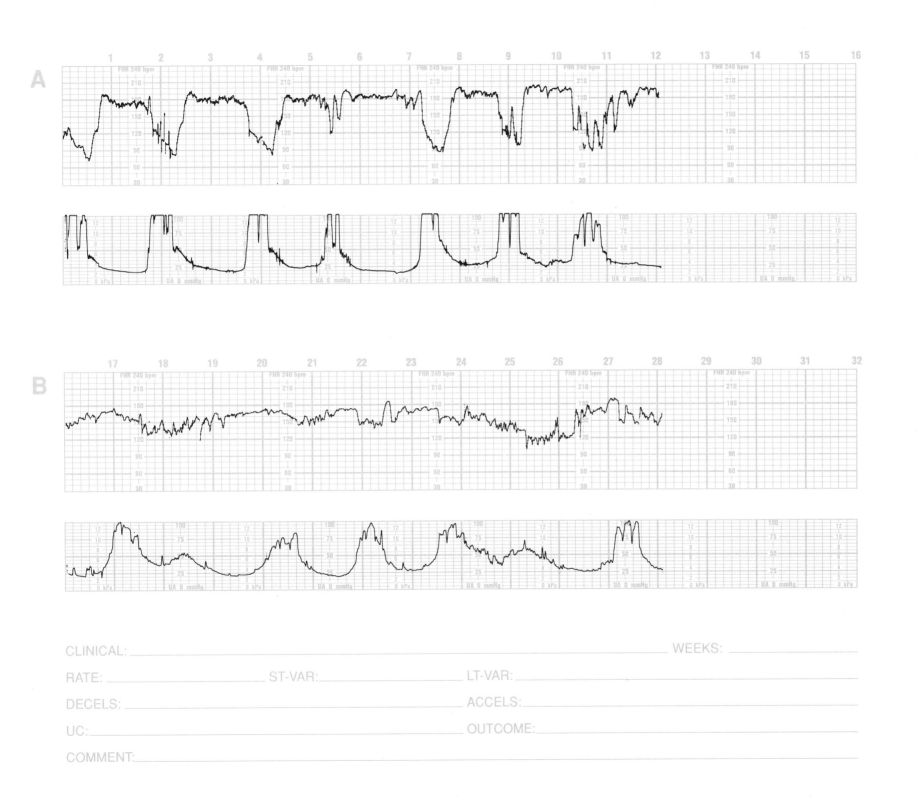

CLINICAL: _____   WEEKS: _____

RATE: _____ ST-VAR: _____   LT-VAR: _____

DECELS: _____   ACCELS: _____

UC: _____   OUTCOME: _____

COMMENT: _____

TRACING: 42

CLINICAL: Normal pregnancy, epidural anesthesia.

WEEKS: Term

BASELINE RATE: 145–160

STV: Decreased, average.

LTV: Decreased, average.

DECELERATIONS: Variable.

ACCELERATIONS: Variable ("shoulders").

UC: Regular—with oxytocin administration (upper); late labor, pushing (lower).

OUTCOME: Normal.

COMMENT: The sentinel deceleration of 13M that appears at 8 cm of cervical dilatation (transition) represents descent of the vertex and is especially common in occiput posterior positions. As in this case, the decelerations continue when the patient starts pushing. The decelerations differ in shape, onset, duration, and amplitude; the angle of the upslope differs as well, as it returns to the baseline. Note especially the decelerations between 23M and 27M. Decelerations with "slow return to baseline," a term that should not be used ("variable deceleration" suffices), generally reveal greater variability than those in which return is more abrupt. Duration of return is of little consequence provided that the prior baseline rate is not exceeded. The geometric pattern at the bottom of the decelerations at 17M, 23M, and thereafter represent arrhythmia. They are variants of nodal or junctional rhythm and do not imply deterioration of the fetal condition. As long as the deceleration returns promptly to the previous baseline rate and variability, neither intervention nor modification of the patient's expulsive efforts is warranted.

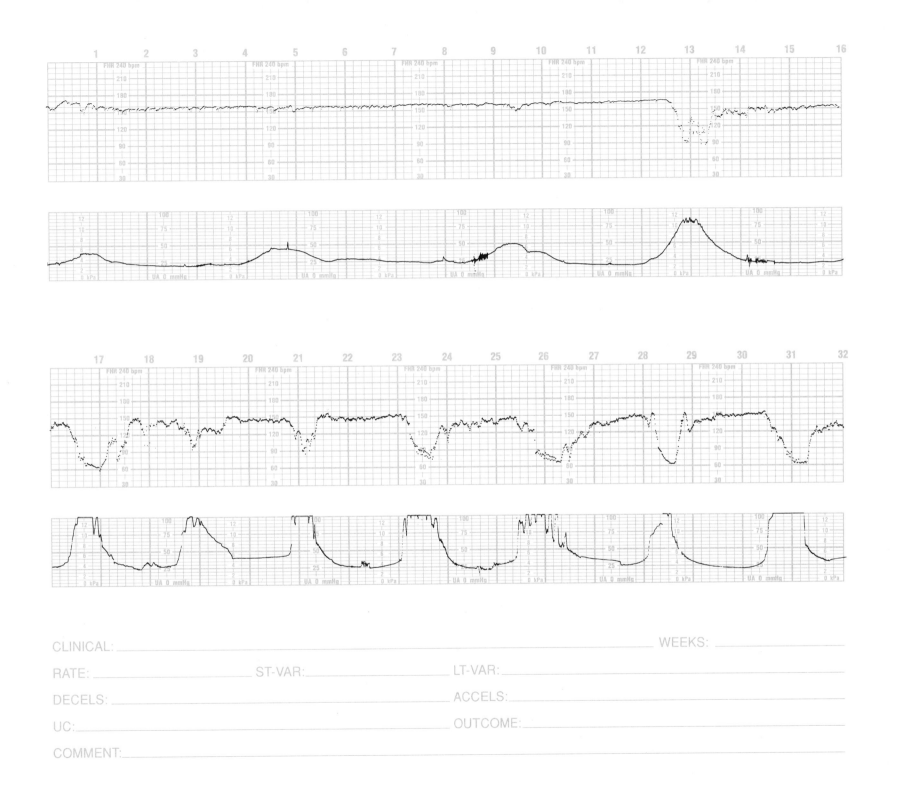

TRACING: 43

CLINICAL: Both: uneventful prenatal course.

WEEKS: Both: 38

BASELINE RATE: Both: 150–160

STV: A: Decreased. B: Average.

LTV: Both: average to increased.

DECELERATIONS: Both: variable.

ACCELERATIONS: Both: variable ("shoulders").

UC: A: Irregular, coupling. B: Second stage.

OUTCOME: Both: Apgar scores, 8/9; uneventful neonatal course.

COMMENT: The *upper panel* reveals a sinusoidal FHR pattern associated with narcotic administration in a particularly susceptible fetus. The sine wave is characteristically 2 to 6 cycles/minute, 5 to 15 bpm in amplitude, and will wax and wane according to the presence of contractions. Notice the occasional variable decelerations with contractions that modulate only slightly the sinusoidal pattern. There is considerable irregularity within the cycles of the sine wave. The preceding tracing was reassuring. Implicitly, this tracing again illustrates the benefit of a baseline tracing prior to the administration of any medication to the mother or fetus. The *lower panel* illustrates larger oscillatory excursions that are sometimes confused with the sinusoidal pattern. These dramatic excursions that occur at the end of variable decelerations are sometimes referred to as saltatory (jumping) or "vagal" patterns. They should not be referred to as "slow return to the baseline." Such changes are seen in resilient (unmedicated) fetuses. These patterns rarely deteriorate. This infant was born with a nuchal cord wrapped twice around the neck.

104

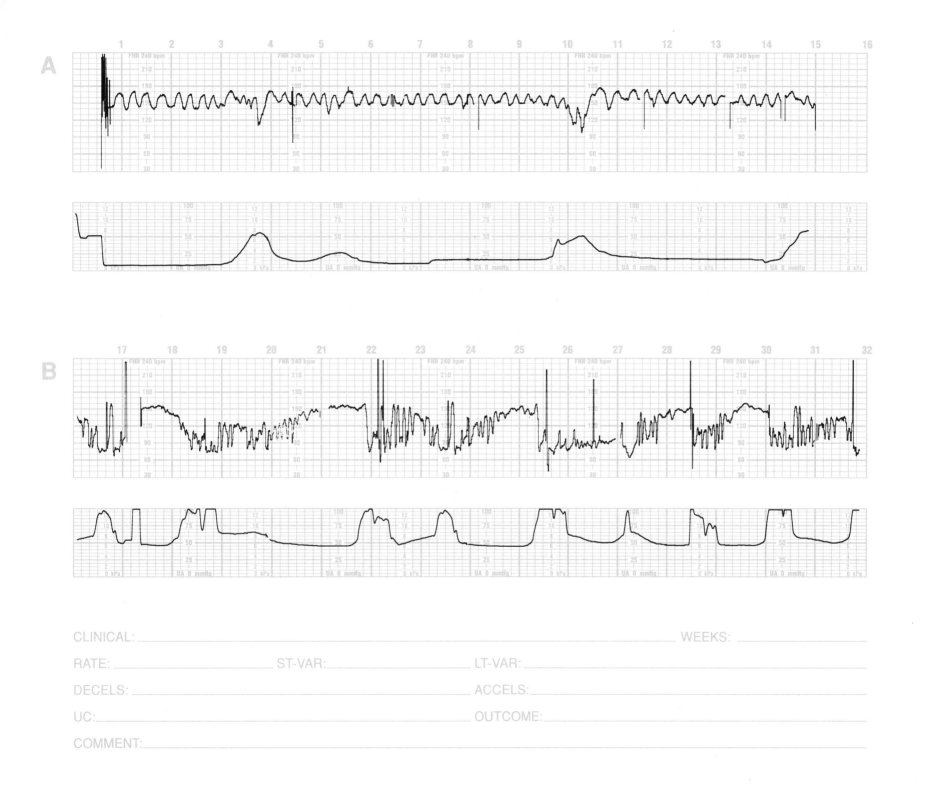

CLINICAL: _____ WEEKS: _____

RATE: _____ ST-VAR: _____ LT-VAR: _____

DECELS: _____ ACCELS: _____

UC: _____ OUTCOME: _____

COMMENT: _____

TRACING: 44

CLINICAL: Uneventful prenatal course.

WEEKS: 41

BASELINE RATE: 150

STV: Average.

LTV: Average.

DECELERATIONS: Variable.

ACCELERATIONS: Variable ("shoulders").

UC: Regular.

OUTCOME: Apgar scores, 9/9; uneventful neonatal course.

COMMENT: The three distinct parts of this tracing derive from the same fetus. The tracing begins with a stable baseline rate, normal variability, and several inconsequential variable decelerations with reasonable recovery. There follows a series of variable decelerations increasing in amplitude and duration and coupling without prompt recovery. These decelerations fail to respond to position changes including Trendelenburg and knee-chest position and vaginal examination fails to reveal an obvious prolapse as cause of the decelerations. The patient was moved to the delivery room at 16M where gentle, manual elevation of the vertex was undertaken while preparations were made for cesarean section. With elevation of the vertex all decelerations disappeared. At that point, several management options were available. First, the physician could make the diagnosis of occult prolapse of the cord while maintaining the vertex in an elevated position and, with other personnel, undertake cesarean section. Alternatively, as in this case, the hand may be removed and the pattern observed at 24M. Ultimately, the patient delivered the infant vaginally with only occasional variable decelerations. No evidence of cord prolapse was found.

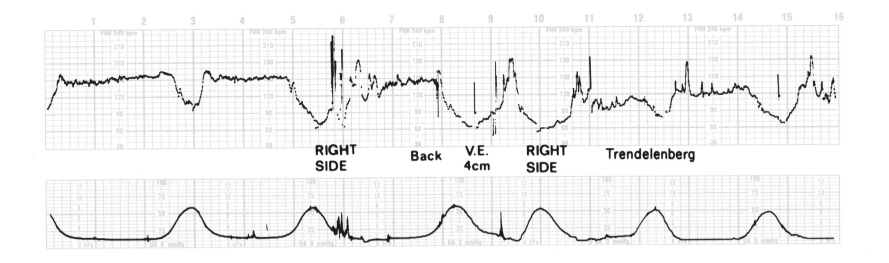

RIGHT SIDE Back V.E. 4cm RIGHT SIDE Trendelenberg

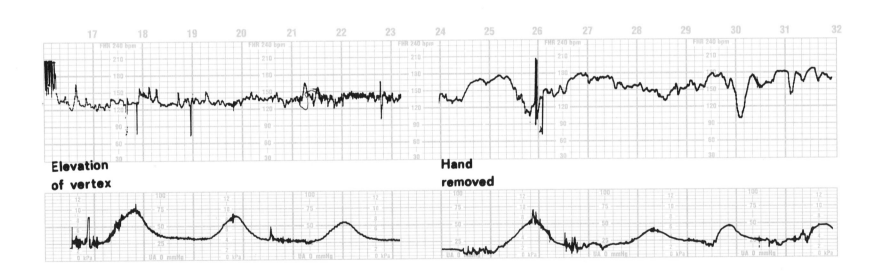

Elevation of vertex

Hand removed

CLINICAL: _____ WEEKS: _____

RATE: _____ ST-VAR: _____ LT-VAR: _____

DECELS: _____ ACCELS: _____

UC: _____ OUTCOME: _____

COMMENT: _____

TRACING: 45

CLINICAL: Uneventful prenatal course.

WEEKS: 39

BASELINE RATE: 130–145

STV: Average.

LTV: Average.

DECELERATIONS: Variable.

ACCELERATIONS: Variable ("shoulders").

UC: Second stage.

OUTCOME: Apgar scores, 8/9; marked moulding; uneventful neonatal course.

COMMENT: This tracing demonstrates the typical FHR pattern associated with occiput-posterior positions during the second stage of labor. The tracing is dominated by recurrent, variable decelerations, some of which reach 60 bpm and develop transient, nodal rhythm (9M, 11M, and 13M). Despite the frequent decelerations and contractions (10 per 16 minutes), the baseline rate remains quite stable without loss of variability. The frequent accelerations ("shoulders") both initiate and follow the decelerations. Fetuses with occiput posterior positions tend to have far more frequent variable decelerations than occiput anteriors, presumably as a result of the increased moulding in this position. The variable decelerations tend to be isolated rather than coalesced and usually return promptly to baseline on cessation of expulsive efforts. No intervention is required here but it is important to restrict expulsive efforts to those times at which the FHR pattern has returned to normal after a previous deceleration.

108

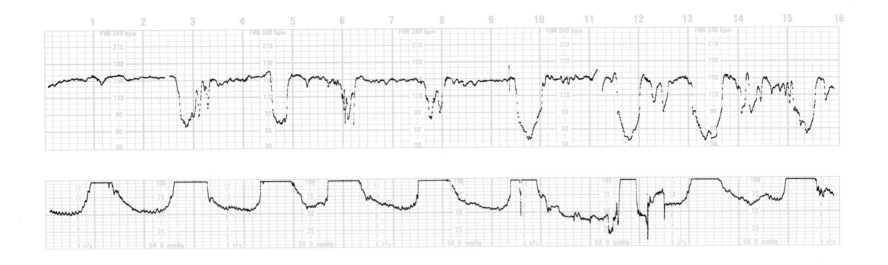

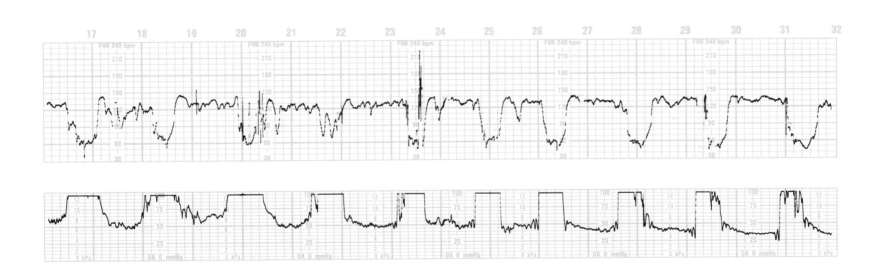

CLINICAL: _____ WEEKS: _____

RATE: _____ ST-VAR: _____ LT-VAR: _____

DECELS: _____ ACCELS: _____

UC: _____ OUTCOME: _____

COMMENT: _____

TRACING: 46

CLINICAL: Uneventful prenatal course.

WEEKS: 40

BASELINE RATE: 130

STV: Average to increased.

LTV: Average to increased.

DECELERATIONS: Variable.

ACCELERATIONS: Variable ("shoulders").

UC: Artifact, second stage.

OUTCOME: Apgar scores, 8/9; unremarkable neonatal course

COMMENT: This tracing illustrates artifact, arrhythmia, and exaggerated variability. The ruler-flat line in the first 10 minutes is artifact. Irrespective of the amounts of narcotic, sedative, or tranquilizer given to the mother, some undulations in the tracing can always be found. Punctuating this line are random, mostly downward excursions in the rate. This pattern develops when the electrode is not applied to the fetus. With proper application at 11M, the tracing reveals a reassuring FHR pattern with normal to increased variability and exaggerated excursions associated with the bearing-down efforts. At 17M, variability diminishes and an arrhythmia appears. Notice the symmetry of these deflections that drop to about half the baseline rate. These represent fetal extrasystoles, erroneously detected to give the appearance of skipped beats. On 5 occasions the actual premature beats are detected properly and represented as excursions that initially extend upward then downward below the baseline followed by a return to the baseline. Without obvious explanation, the pattern then returns to the earlier, more dramatic, decelerative pattern. Although the fetus spends most of its time decelerating, it maintains normal, if not exaggerated, variability with the occasional premature beats. Contractions are coming every 1 to 1½ minutes with considerable artifact in the first 10 minutes. The transducer, positioned improperly, lifts off the patient's abdomen during bearing-down efforts. This produces the initial, upward deflection, immediately followed by an equally abrupt downward deflection. The transducer is repositioned at about 8M, revealing a customary contraction pattern.

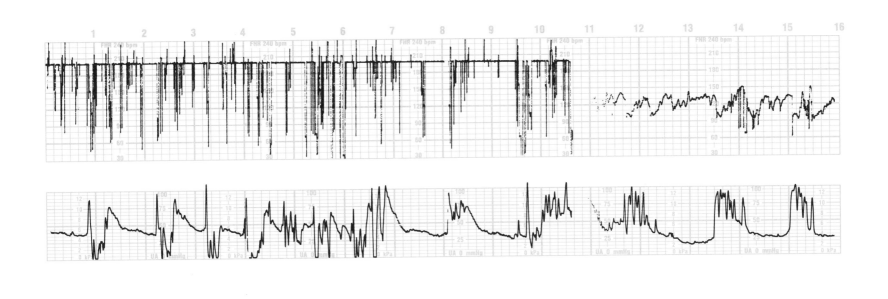

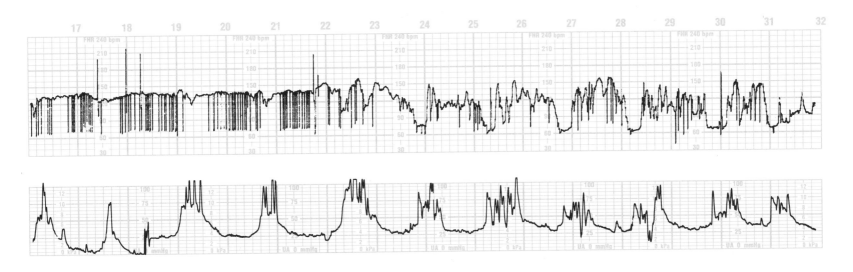

TRACING: 47

CLINICAL: Uneventful prenatal course.

WEEKS: 41

BASELINE RATE: 140

STV: Average.

LTV: Average to increased.

DECELERATIONS: Variable.

ACCELERATIONS: Variable ("shoulders").

UC: Second stage.

OUTCOME: Apgar scores, 7/8; uneventful neonatal course.

COMMENT: This tracing illustrates frequent, variable decelerations with "slow return to the baseline." Despite the very frequent contractions and decelerations, the baseline heart rate remains stable with satisfactory and sometimes increased variability (saltatory pattern). These dramatic changes are quite frequent during the second stage especially in uncomplicated labors. They frequently, but not always, moderate when pushing ceases. In this case, cessation of pushing, if anything, exaggerates the saltatory pattern. Saltatory ("vagal") patterns suggest compensation for previous episodes of stress, but probably not asphyxial stress. Intervention is unnecessary in this case and deterioration is uncommon.

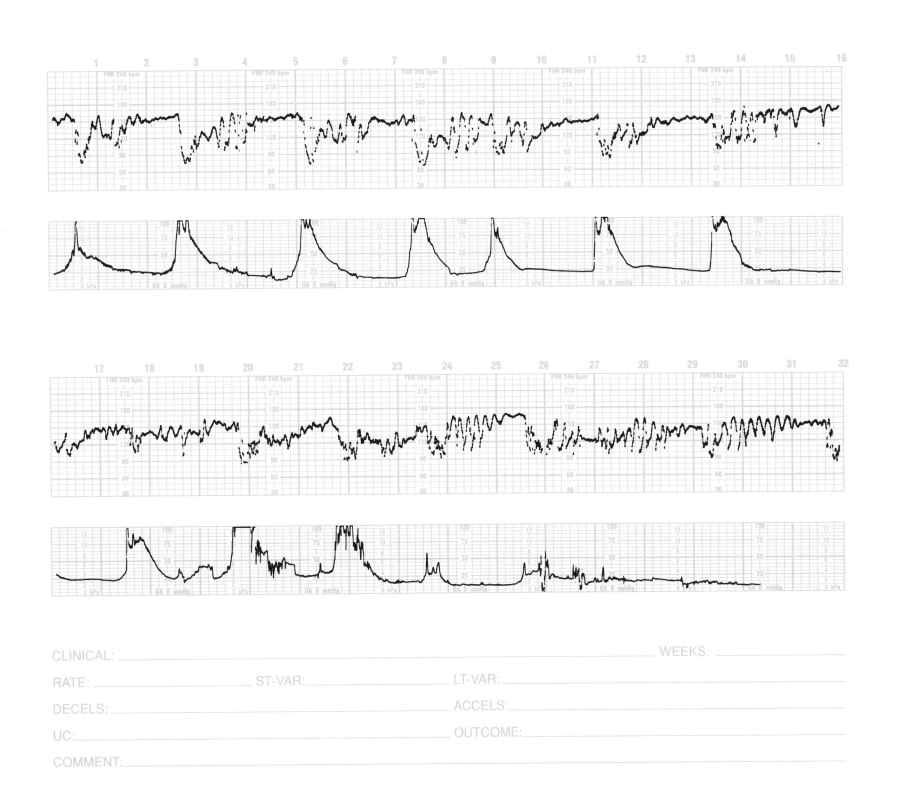

TRACING: 48

CLINICAL: Normal pregnancy, late labor.

WEEKS: 39

BASELINE RATE: 170, decreases toward end.

STV: Average.

LTV: Average.

DECELERATIONS: Late or variable?

ACCELERATIONS: None.

UC: Late labor, expulsive efforts.

OUTCOME: Normal Apgar scores.

COMMENT: This tracing is included for those who cannot make up their minds. If you wish to argue these are late decelerations, you might offer the following: These are relatively uniform, recurrent decelerations that tend to arise late in the contraction cycle, returning to baseline after the contraction is over. If you maintain that these are variable decelerations you might argue as follows: While these decelerations have all the characteristics described above, we nevertheless find some inconsistency in the relationship between the amplitude of the decelerations and the amplitude of the associated contractions. These very frequent contractions and associated expulsive efforts clearly induce decelerations but, if anything, the baseline rate is declining rather than rising, and normal baseline variability is maintained. In addition, the decelerations appear only after the onset of pushing. These arguments speak against the decelerations being late decelerations. Note the discrepancy between the onset of the decelerations and the onset of the contractions at 5M and 30M. Also note the small arrhythmias at 23M and 26M+ (more common with variable decelerations).

Which argument do you prefer? Would cessation of pushing resolve the argument? Clue: look at the beginning of the tracing. Which position do you think the baby is in (occiput anterior, or posterior)? Do you think this baby will deliver vaginally? Why? If you believe that these are late decelerations, would you consider it a failure of the standard of care if someone else called them variable decelerations?

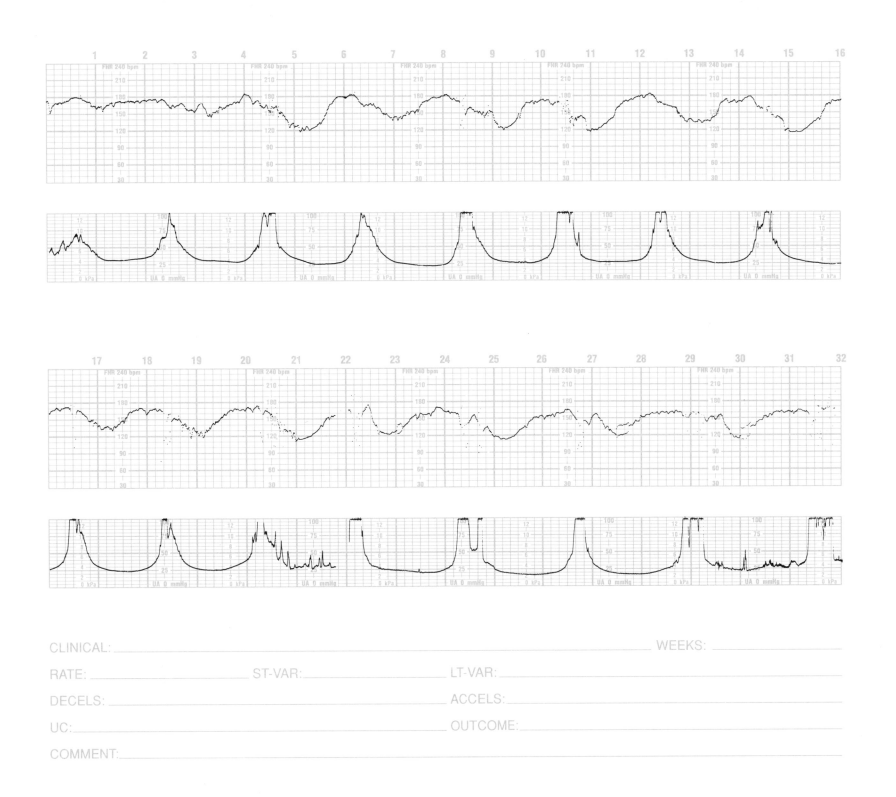

TRACING: 49

CLINICAL: A: Premature labor, hypertension, IUGR. B: Uneventful prenatal course.

WEEKS: A: 33. B: 40.

BASELINE RATE: A: 160. B: 150.

STV: A: Absent. B: Average.

LTV: A: Absent. B: Average.

DECELERATIONS: A: Variable, late. B: Variable.

ACCELERATIONS: A: Overshoot. B: Variable ("shoulders").

UC: A: By palpation. B: Second stage.

OUTCOME: A: Apgar scores, 0/3; neonatal death. B: Apgar scores, 7/9; uneventful neonatal course.

COMMENT: The *upper* and *lower panels* represent different fetuses. The *upper panel* presents a most ominous heart rate pattern in a premature infant. Here, recurrent, combined variable/late decelerations accompany each contraction as determined by palpation. Notice the attempt of the baseline to rise following each coupled deceleration. Despite the obvious compromise, the variable decelerations are rarely prolonged. The baby delivered shortly thereafter and died in the neonatal period.

In the *lower panel,* secondary decelerations (which manifest no obvious pattern) follow immediately upon obvious variable decelerations and their accompanying variable accelerations ("shoulders"). Sometimes the shoulders are high and spiked, sometimes broad. The secondary decelerations at 15M, 29M, and 31M should not be considered as late or combined variable/late decelerations. They are inconstant in appearance and shape, and bear no obvious relationship to the preceding deceleration. Indeed, the largest deceleration, at 24M, is not followed by a secondary deceleration. The variation in the recovery pattern of the deceleration and the ability of the baby to maintain variability is clearly a function of adequate reserve.

116

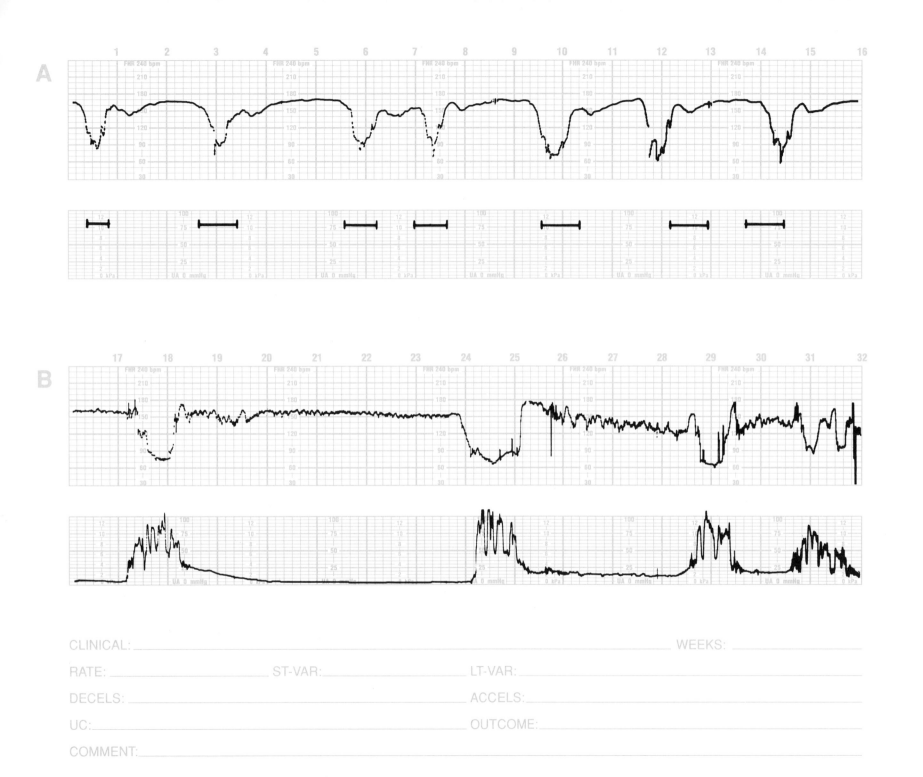

TRACING: 50

CLINICAL: Preterm labor.

WEEKS: 35

BASELINE RATE: 160

STV: Absent.

LTV: Absent.

DECELERATIONS: Late.

ACCELERATIONS: None.

UC: Regular.

OUTCOME: Apgar scores, 1/2; meconium staining; cesarean section; neonatal death.

COMMENT: This tracing illustrates the potential pitfall in assessing variability from external transducers. Both *upper* and *lower panels* derive from the same fetus. In the *upper* tracing the ultrasound transducer introduces extraneous variability while in the *lower* tracing, the direct electrode reveals the absent variability. Recurrent decelerations are obvious in both panels but the impression of baseline variability differs dramatically in the two. The detection of decelerations with the external device requires direct monitoring, if feasible.

This tracing is quite ominous, revealing a combination of acute distress, late decelerations, and chronic distress with a flat heart rate baseline and slight tachycardia. Immediate preparations for delivery are required. While conservative maneuvers such as oxygen, lateral position, and hydration are appropriate, they are unlikely to ameliorate the fetal condition. Oxygen may reduce or eliminate the late decelerations but not improve the fetal condition. Before deciding to continue with the labor, oxygen should be discontinued. If decelerations reappear and contraindications are absent, the fetus should be delivered expeditiously. If decelerations do not reappear after oxygen removal then the acute distress has been alleviated and an intelligent decision must be made about the chronic distress pattern.

The findings on this tracing preclude the explanation that the tracing was "normal 5 minutes earlier" and that earlier intervention in this case would have made a difference in the outcome. Given the stable baseline rate and absent variability, we may reasonably infer that the monitoring was begun long after the onset of asphyxia.

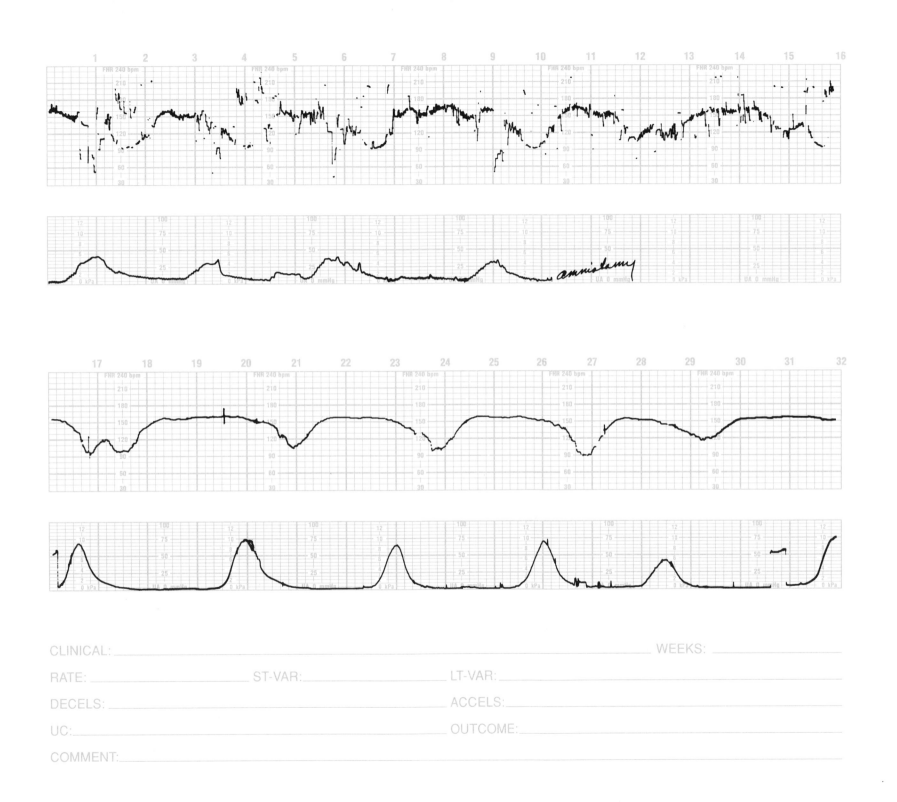

amniotamy

CLINICAL: _____ WEEKS: _____

RATE: _____ ST-VAR: _____ LT-VAR: _____

DECELS: _____ ACCELS: _____

UC: _____ OUTCOME: _____

COMMENT: _____

TRACING: 51

CLINICAL: Severe hypertension, growth retardation.

WEEKS: 34

BASELINE RATE: 150–160

STV: Absent.

LTV: Absent.

DECELERATIONS: Recurrent lates, some variable.

ACCELERATIONS: Occasional overshoot.

UC: Recurrent, coupled contractions, oxytocin effect.

OUTCOME: Apgar scores, 2/4; respiratory distress syndrome.

COMMENT: This ominous tracing reveals absent variability and late decelerations (1M, 5M+, 11M–16M, etc.). Occasionally some of the late decelerations are overwhelmed by variable decelerations (4M, 8M+, 19M, etc.). The variable decelerations are best defined by the slope and amplitude and presence of nodal rhythm at the nadir of the deceleration. The distinction between late and variable decelerations at this advanced stage of distress is of little consequence. The tracing demanded aggressive care long before this.

The dramatic change in the appearance of the tracing at 17M results from the change in paper speed from 3 to 1 cm/minute while the vertical scaling is maintained at 30 bpm/cm. The effect of this change in the "aspect ratio" compresses the decelerations, modifies their appearance, creates confusion in the identification of the individual deceleration and invites the suggestion that the decelerations are coupled (e.g., 22M). In ad-

dition, slowing the paper speed increases the amount of apparent variability.

The tracings in this book represent a reduction to 45% of the original. They remain recognizable because of the simultaneous reduction of both the horizontal and the vertical axes. The proportion of vertical height to horizontal width is referred to as the "aspect ratio." As long as the aspect ratio is kept constant, the pattern remains recognizable irrespective of reduction or enlargement. When the paper speed is changed, from 3 to 1 cm or vice versa, the horizontal axis is modified, but not the vertical axis. As a result, the aspect ratio is modified and the pattern is less recognizable. There is no virtue to one speed or scaling factor over another—the choice should be predicated on an individual's training and experience. Most tracings published in the United States use the 3 cm/minute, 30 bpm/cm scaling factors.

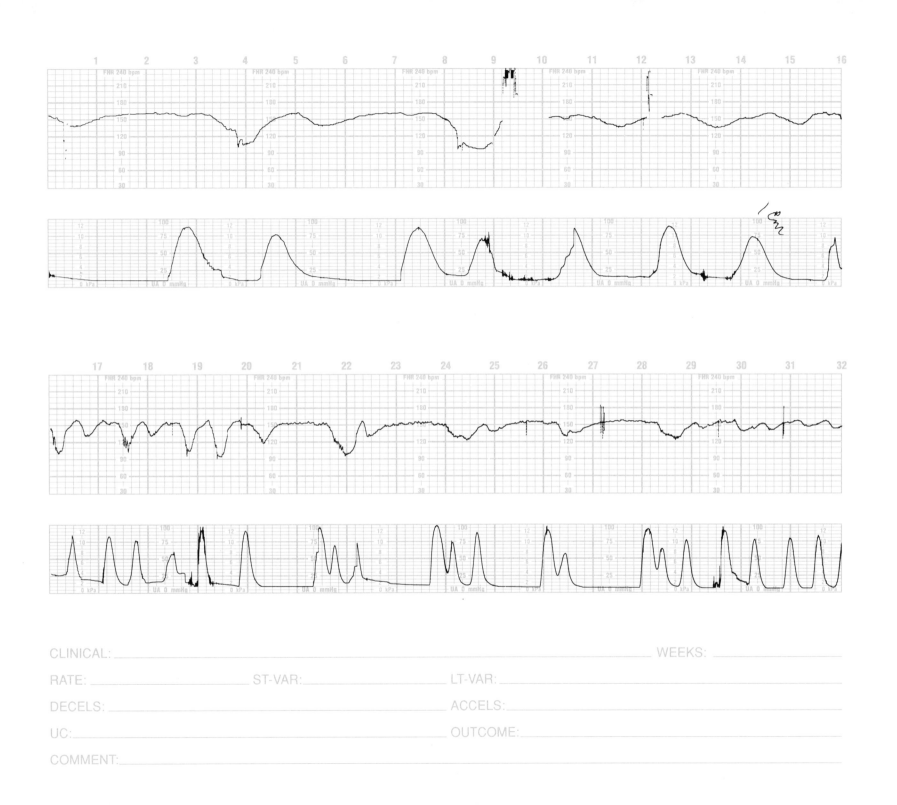

CLINICAL: _____   WEEKS: _____

RATE: _____ ST-VAR: _____   LT-VAR: _____

DECELS: _____   ACCELS: _____

UC: _____   OUTCOME: _____

COMMENT: _____

TRACING: 52

CLINICAL: Postdates.

WEEKS: 42

BASELINE RATE: 140

STV: Absent.

LTV: Absent.

DECELERATIONS: Late.

ACCELERATIONS: None.

UC: Occasional, not in labor.

OUTCOME: Apgar scores, 0/1; cesarean section; neonatal hematocrit 10%; fetal-maternal transfusion; neonatal death.

COMMENT: This is an ominous FHR pattern consisting of absent variability and recurrent late decelerations despite infrequent contractions. The first 4 minutes of FHR pattern are obtained with an ultrasound transducer that characteristically exaggerates the amount of variability. The change from external transducer to internal electrode reveals the dramatic difference. The artifact at 5M should not be confused with arrhythmia. This reflects the electronic distortion introduced by the monitor as it attempts to optimize the fetal signal for counting. Notice the episodes of minuscule, beat-to-beat arrhythmia (bigeminy) at 12M, 21M, and just before 32M during the recovery from the decelerations.

These could never be detected by external transducers. These beat-to-beat arrhythmias suggest an accumulation of carbon dioxide with elaboration of catecholamines. There is a small, late deceleration at 14M. At this stage of compromise, the certain distinction between late and variable decelerations is important.

This patient presented at 42 weeks' gestation for induction of labor. Rupture of the membranes revealed bloody amniotic fluid. Immediate cesarean section produced a hopelessly asphyxiated, pale infant with a hematocrit of 10%, who subsequently died. Kleihauer-Betke examination of the maternal blood drawn before the operation revealed a large fetal-maternal transfusion.

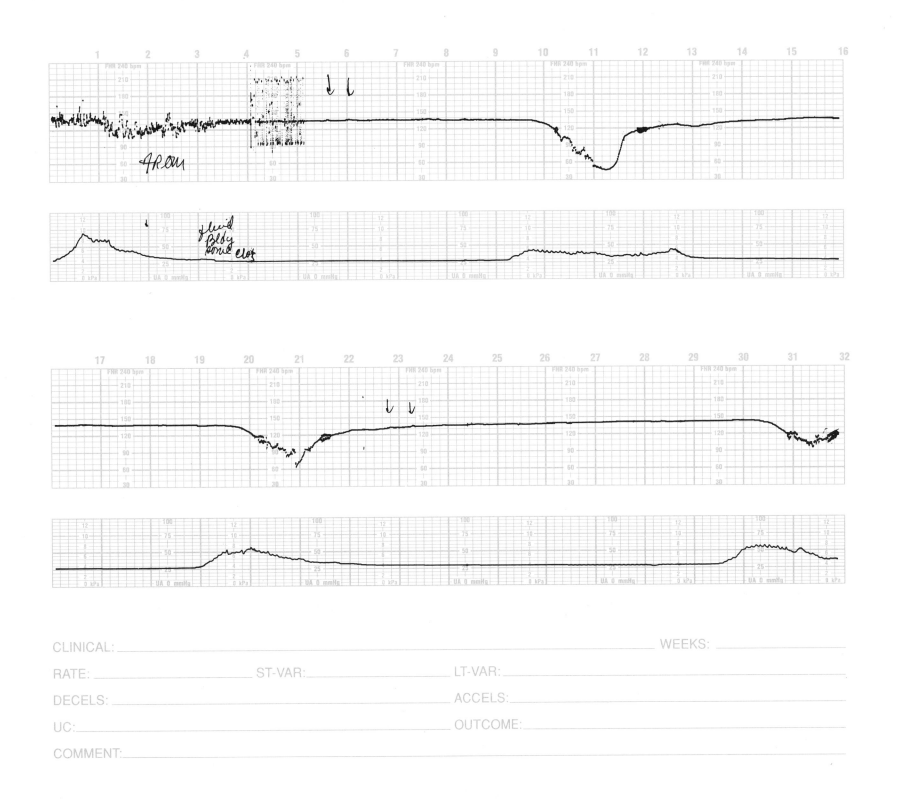

CLINICAL: _____ WEEKS: _____

RATE: _____ ST-VAR: _____ LT-VAR: _____

DECELS: _____ ACCELS: _____

UC: _____ OUTCOME: _____

COMMENT: _____

TRACING: 53

CLINICAL: Normal labor.

WEEKS: 38

BASELINE RATE: 170 to 180

STV: Average.

LTV: Average.

DECELERATIONS: Recurrent variable.

ACCELERATIONS: None.

UC: Late labor, pushing with contractions.

OUTCOME: Apgar scores, 1, 6, and 8.

COMMENT: This tracing reveals the risks to the fetus of unrestrained expulsive efforts with an occiput posterior position. The tracing reveals recurrent, variable decelerations. Despite their depth, duration, tendency to produce transient asystole, and recovery to an elevated baseline rate, they require conservative management, not intervention. The baseline rate, though elevated, is quite stable and reveals reasonable variability. The decelerations begin abruptly, reach a nadir rapidly, and return promptly to the previous baseline without overshoot. Only the first two decelerations contain transient episodes of cardiac asystole at the base, the remainder do not. These episodes induce no obvious changes in the return to the baseline rate or in the baseline variability when compared to the other decelerations. The apparent deceleration at 6M, seemingly a late deceleration, may be discounted. No other contraction either before or after re-peats the same phenomenon. It may be related to the excessive variability after the preceding variable deceleration.

A vaginal examination during the deceleration at 13M induces a prolonged deceleration. Because the patient is in the second stage of labor she is encouraged to push, which only maintains the slow rate. When pushing is stopped transiently, the rate begins to recover although it does not reach the previous rate (18M–19M). Immediately thereafter, pushing is reinstituted (more obvious with the repositioned transducer); the FHR starts down, reaches about 60 bpm, and reenters nodal rhythm with absent variability. Despite the low, flat heart rate, the trend over the next minute is ever-so-slightly upward (22M–23M). The patient is removed to the delivery room at 24M, where the low rate and absent variability are confirmed. Notice that now the nodal rhythm is headed downward. This is a most ominous sign that anticipates fetal death without prompt intervention.

This life-threatening sequence is more common when the occiput is posterior and when the patient's expulsive efforts are sustained in the presence of an abnormal FHR pattern. Ordinarily, when decelerations accompany expulsive efforts, cessation of pushing allows the heart rate to recover. If there is delay in the return, pushing must be discouraged until the FHR has recovered to its previous baseline rate and variability.

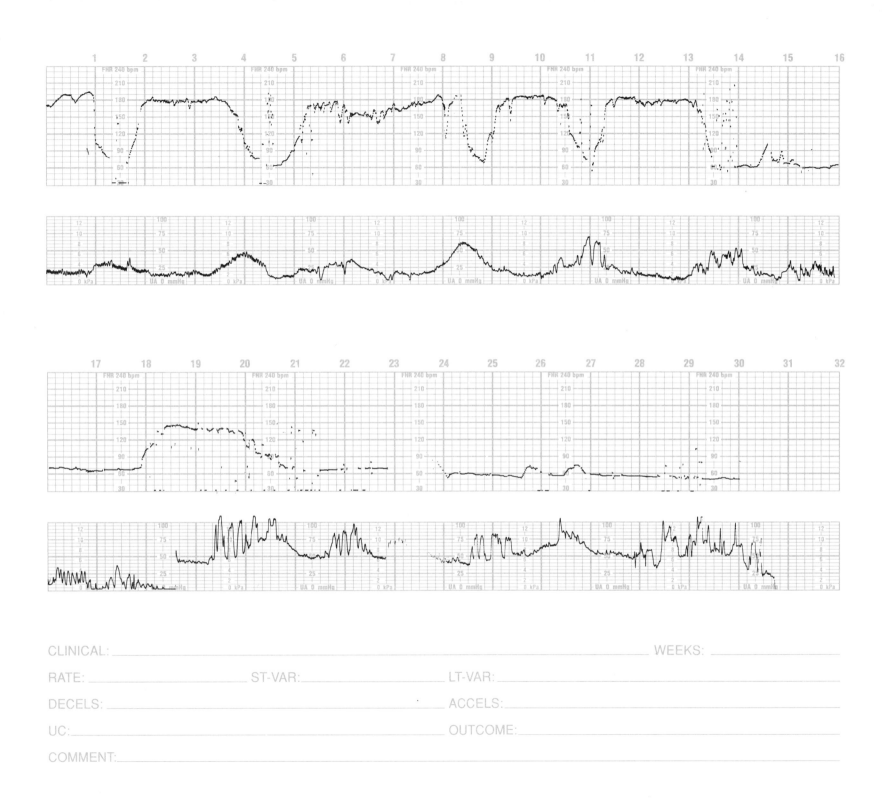

CLINICAL: _____ WEEKS: _____

RATE: _____ ST-VAR: _____ LT-VAR: _____

DECELS: _____ ACCELS: _____

UC: _____ OUTCOME: _____

COMMENT: _____

TRACING: 54

CLINICAL: Uneventful prenatal course.

WEEKS: 41

BASELINE RATE: 150

STV: Average.

LTV: Average.

DECELERATIONS: Variable, prolonged.

ACCELERATIONS: Variable ("shoulders").

UC: Second stage.

OUTCOME: Apgar scores, 9/9; cesarean section; occult cord prolapse, uneventful neonatal course.

COMMENT: This tracing reveals characteristic decelerations during the second stage of labor that progress to a life-threatening situation. The fetus is in occiput-transverse position. The combination of frequent uterine contractions and relentless pushing with contractions induces a series of variable decelerations (anyone for lates?) that evolve into a prolonged, sustained deceleration. Several contractions without expulsive efforts (22M, 25M) produce either no further deceleration or at least attempted recovery. The resumption of pushing perpetuates the downward trend of the heart rate. Because pushing with contractions enhances the risk of both mechanical and hypoxemic stress, cessation of pushing may have profound salutary effects on the FHR patterns of the second stage. In this case, the patient was taken immediately to the operating room where the vertex was elevated and the FHR returned promptly to about 140 bpm.

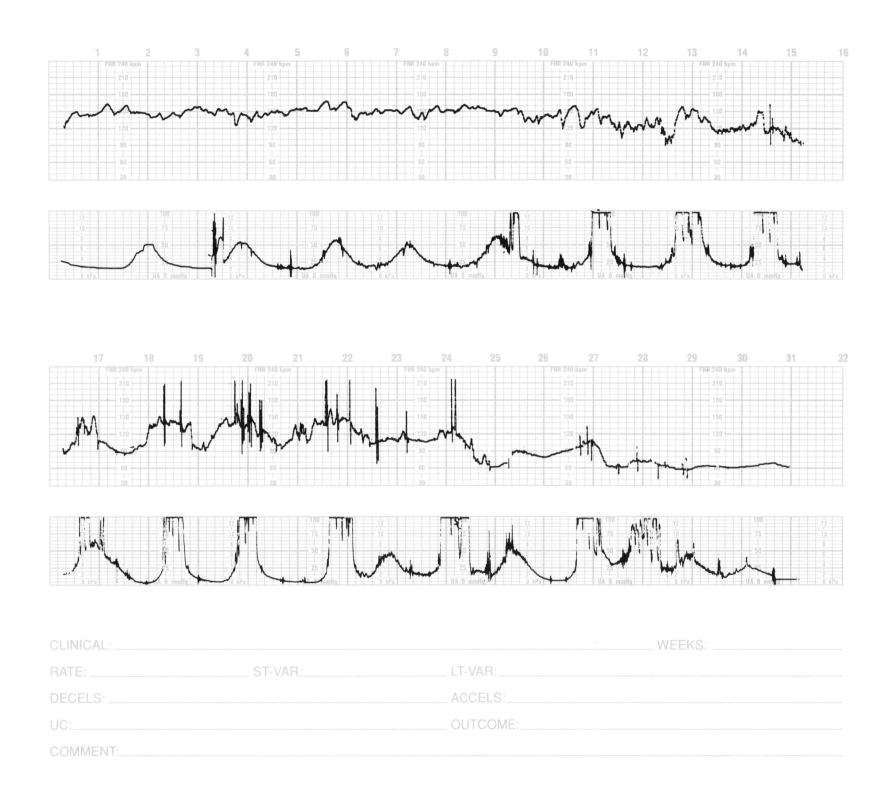

TRACING: 55

CLINICAL: Preterm labor.

WEEKS: 34

BASELINE RATE: 150–160, unstable.

STV: Absent.

LTV: Decreased.

DECELERATIONS: Variable.

ACCELERATIONS: Overshoot.

UC: Late spontaneous labor, baseline changes with position change.

OUTCOME: Low Apgar score, severe respiratory distress.

COMMENT: This disturbing pattern contains variable decelerations with overshoot irrespective of the amplitude of the deceleration. The tracing also reveals a small area of sinusoidal oscillations at the beginning of the tracing. Except for the single, deep variable deceleration at 20M the remaining decelerations are trivial and do not bespeak significant asphyxia related to cord compression.

Ominous sinusoidal patterns are usually *not* persistent and preclude normal variability elsewhere. Often they appear along with absent (short-term) variability after variable decelerations or without a deceleration at the end of the contraction (when you would expect a late deceleration).

This pattern with the relatively high baseline rate is consistent with injury, anomaly, prematurity, or atropine administration. The temptation to identify the small decelerations at 13M,

23M, and 26M as early decelerations should be resisted. Benign, early decelerations are proportional in amplitude and duration to the amplitude and duration of the underlying contraction. By definition, they do not show trailing accelerations (overshoot). When these decelerations are seen during antepartum testing (with a nonreactive NST) they have been referred to as "atypical" (see Freeman RK, James J: Clinical experience with the oxytocin challenge test: II. An ominous atypical pattern. *Obstet Gynecol* 1977; 46:255).

Although there is no significant acute distress in this tracing, the potential for long-term neurological handicap is considerable. Should this patient undergo cesarean section if immediate delivery is not forseen? This question applies to patients with similar tracings elsewhere in this volume. There is no right answer. Those who believe that no intervention is indicated may justify their decision (in a reasoned note) as follows: Although this pattern provokes great concern about the potential for subsequent neurologic handicap, there is no obvious acute distress or evidence of deterioration. In the absence of decelerations there is no evidence that cesarean section will make a difference in outcome. Given the potential for the development of fetal distress, however, the patient has been prepared for cesarean section should the need arise.

Those who find cesarean section appealing might argue (in their well-reasoned note) as follows: This chronic pattern provokes great concern for the ultimate neurologic outcome of the fetus. Although there is no obvious acute fetal distress at present, the potential for such an eventuality is increased with such patterns. These considerations suggest that cesarean section at this time is a most reasonable strategy. Which strategy do you prefer? Which one is right?

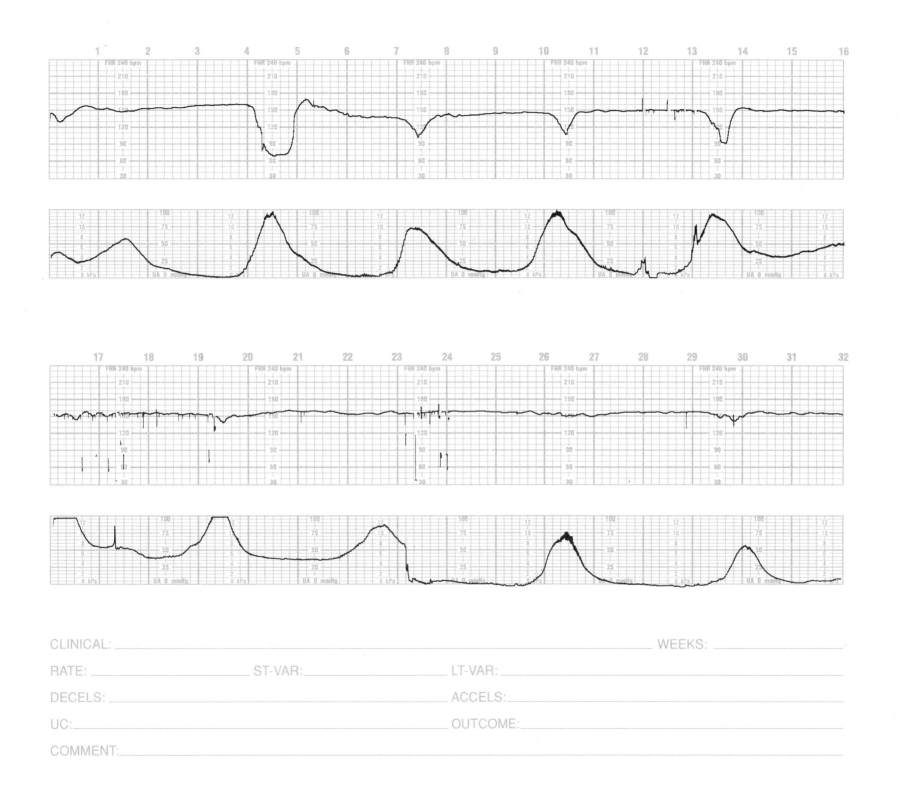

CLINICAL: _____ WEEKS: _____

RATE: _____ ST-VAR: _____ LT-VAR: _____

DECELS: _____ ACCELS: _____

UC: _____ OUTCOME: _____

COMMENT: _____

TRACING: 56

CLINICAL: Oligohydramnios.

WEEKS: 42

BASELINE RATE: 150–155

STV: Absent.

LTV: Absent.

DECELERATIONS: Brief variables.

ACCELERATIONS: Overshoot.

UC: Advanced labor.

OUTCOME: Low Apgar scores, neurologic handicap.

COMMENT: Despite the absence of any dramatic changes, this unique pattern offers considerable insight into the signs of neurologic abnormality in the fetus. The entire pattern takes place in the second stage of labor; contractions are frequent and the mother is pushing with each. Despite this assault, the fetus maintains a perfectly stable baseline rate with some accelerations and no decelerations—features that preclude fetal asphyxia. For the skeptical, this is confirmed in the *lower panel* with normal fetal scalp pH samples of 7.28 and 7.26. While superficial scanning suggests the contractions are associated with fetal cardiac accelerations, closer inspection shows that most accelerations are anticipated by slight decelerations or notches—at 2M, 4M, 10M, and 14M. In the *lower panel* they are more representative of small variable decelerations with overshoot—at 18M, 21M, 23M, 26M, and 30M. In these examples, the acceleration is usually larger than the preceding deceleration.

In the normal fetus, accelerations usually arise from normal baseline variability without premonitory decelerations. This pattern suggests autonomic imbalance. In the absence of atropine, other drugs, or immaturity, one must consider the potential for neurologic abnormality secondary to congenital anomaly or prior insult.

The questions of management are discussed in tracing 55. How would you interpret this pattern if this were a non-stress test, and the heart rate pattern were being obtained with ultrasound? Under these circumstances the variability would be artificially exaggerated and the small premonitory decelerations would be camouflaged by the artifact, leaving only the accelerations.

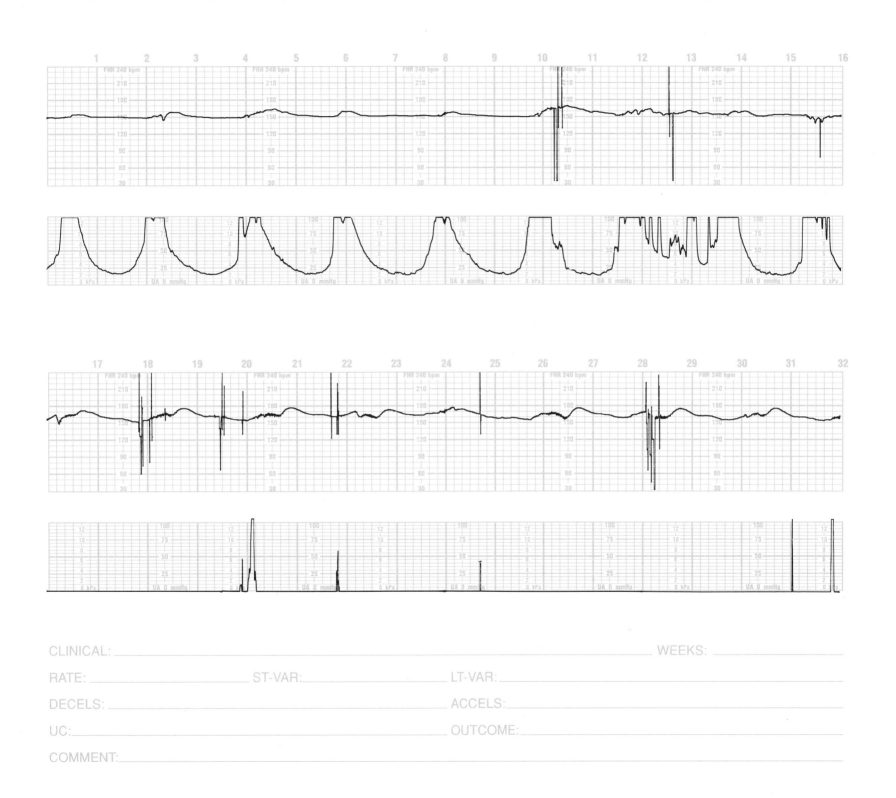

CLINICAL: _____   WEEKS: _____

RATE: _____ ST-VAR: _____ LT-VAR: _____

DECELS: _____ ACCELS: _____

UC: _____ OUTCOME: _____

COMMENT: _____

TRACING: 57

CLINICAL: Postdates, decreased fetal movement.

WEEKS: 43

BASELINE RATE: 180

STV: Absent.

LTV: Absent.

DECELERATIONS: Variable.

ACCELERATIONS: "Overshoot".

UC: Second stage, artifact.

OUTCOME: Apgar scores, 2/6; meconium staining; neonatal seizures; cerebral palsy.

COMMENT: This tracing reveals a chronic heart rate pattern during the second stage of labor. Notice the stable baseline rate, absent variability, and frequent variable decelerations with overshoot. The apparent increase in variability associated with maternal pushing is almost certainly artifact. On the other hand, the small decelerations and accelerations associated with the individual expulsive efforts are certainly real. There is also considerable artifact and blunting of the uterine contraction channel. It has not been well calibrated and does not reflect the excursions in the mother's breathing at all. The abrupt, angulated upslopes of the uterine contractions are quite unphysiologic, suggesting a plugged catheter.

With imminent vaginal delivery, this stable but abnormal tracing presents few management problems. Scalp sampling usually confirms normal pH values. Nevertheless, the potential, but not the inevitability, of untoward outcome must be understood.

At delivery, this meconium-stained, postdate fetus presented with typical features of postmaturity syndrome. The cord blood gases revealed no acidosis. The infant had a seizure within 24 hours and was subsequently found to have cerebral palsy.

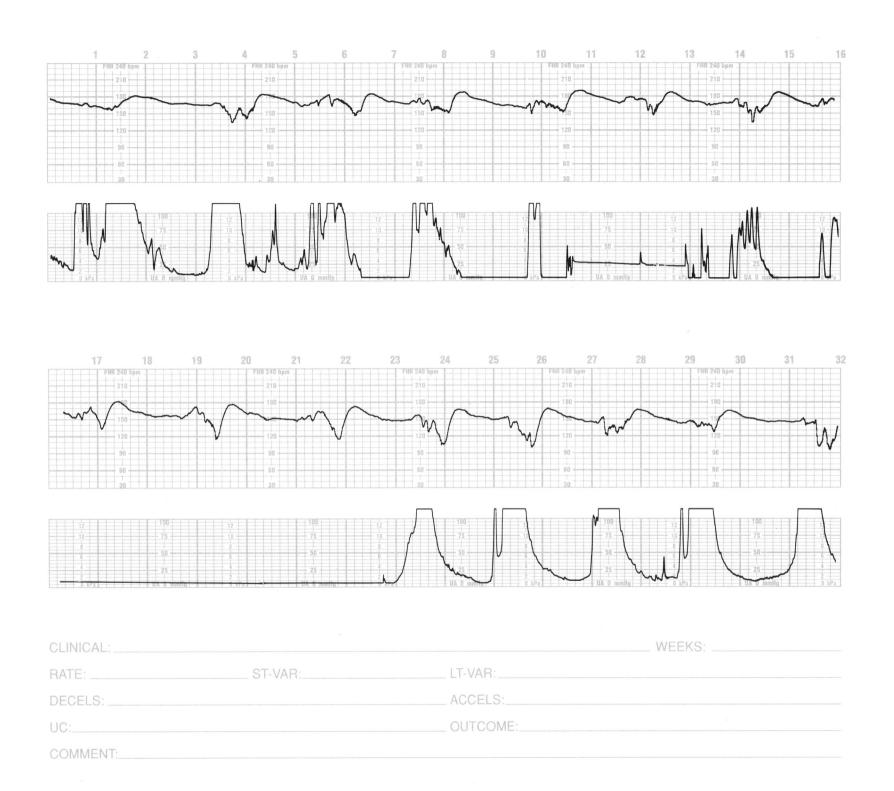

CLINICAL: _____ WEEKS: _____

RATE: _____ ST-VAR: _____ LT-VAR: _____

DECELS: _____ ACCELS: _____

UC: _____ OUTCOME: _____

COMMENT: _____

TRACING: 58

CLINICAL: Uneventful prenatal course, decreased fetal movement.

WEEKS: 39

BASELINE RATE: 180

STV: Absent.

LTV: Absent.

DECELERATIONS: Mild variable.

ACCELERATIONS: "Overshoot."

UC: Infrequent, coupled.

OUTCOME: Apgar scores, 0/0; stillborn.

COMMENT: This tracing illustrates a chronically affected fetus. This is a markedly abnormal FHR pattern, consisting of baseline tachycardia, absent variability, small variable decelerations with overshoot, and some instability of the heart rate as reflected by the prolonged return to the baseline after the occasional contraction. These ongoing features make it implausible that the tracing immediately preceding this could have been normal—to wit: For all the abnormalities in this tracing, the changes are hardly dramatic. Although the fetus has been suffering from asphyxia for quite some time, the infrequent contractions have permitted the infant to deteriorate slowly with only minimal decelerations now that it is so severely compromised. This fetus suffered from a true knot in the cord and died later in labor.

The management implications of this tracing are far from clear. Presumably, prompt cesarean section would have prevented the later stillbirth but it is highly unlikely that the infant would have survived the neonatal period and even less likely that it would have survived intact. Cesarean section carries risks for the mother and does not clearly improve outcome in fetuses with this heart rate pattern.

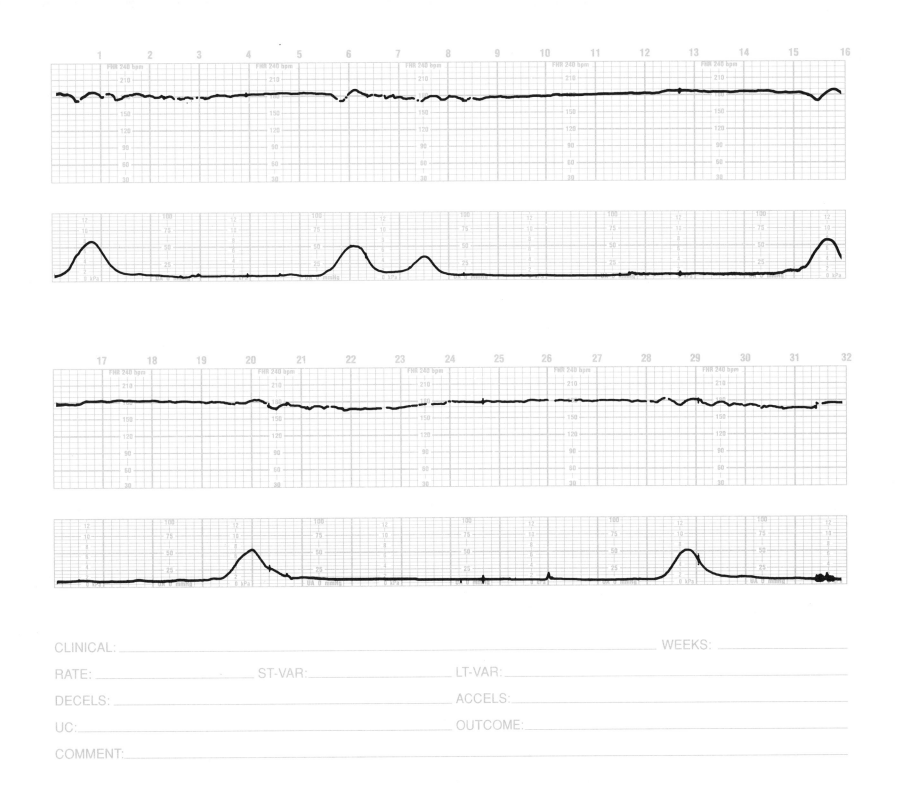

CLINICAL: _____ WEEKS: _____

RATE: _____ ST-VAR: _____ LT-VAR: _____

DECELS: _____ ACCELS: _____

UC: _____ OUTCOME: _____

COMMENT: _____

TRACING: 59

CLINICAL: Hypertension, IUGR, oligohydramnios.

WEEKS: 36

BASELINE RATE: 150

STV: Absent.

LTV: Absent.

DECELERATIONS: Mild variable.

ACCELERATIONS: Rebound ("overshoot").

UC: Regular.

OUTCOME: Apgar scores, 3/6; neonatal seizures; residual neurologic deficit.

COMMENT: This FHR pattern of chronic distress reveals absent variability, and small variable decelerations with overshoot without any consequential late or variable decelerations—no acute distress. In this circumstance, the decision to intervene is unlikely to change the prognosis in any significant way. About one third of these babies may develop acute fetal distress later on in labor, for which cesarean section may be indicated. Those who would argue for cesarean section might cite the potential for developing acute distress and the prevention of any additional harm. Those who opt not to perform cesarean section might resort to scalp sampling, which will probably be normal. They might argue that since there is no acute (asphyxial) distress at the present time, they will prepare for cesarean section but reserve its performance for subsequent developments. There is no right answer—there is only the option for an intelligent choice.

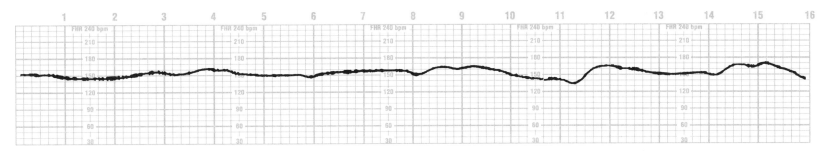

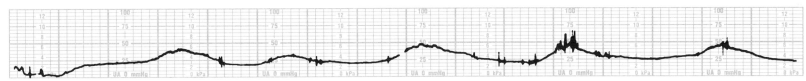

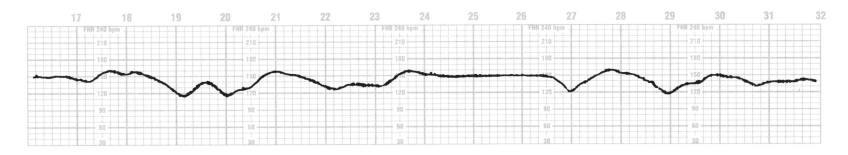

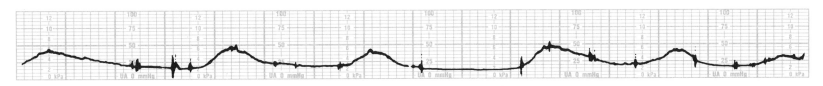

CLINICAL:_____ WEEKS:_____

RATE:_____ ST-VAR:_____ LT-VAR:_____

DECELS:_____ ACCELS:_____

UC:_____ OUTCOME:_____

COMMENT:_____

TRACING: 60

CLINICAL: Oligohydramnios, nonreactive NST.

WEEKS: 41

BASELINE RATE: 125

STV: Absent.

LTV: Absent.

DECELERATIONS: Variable, late.

ACCELERATIONS: Rebound ("overshoot").

UC: Early labor.

OUTCOME: Apgar scores, 2/4; cesarean section; neonatal seizures; meconium aspiration; residual handicap.

COMMENT: This tracing has been introduced here because of its enormous potential for misinterpretation. The first 8 minutes are obtained by external ultrasound transducer and we see the characteristic exaggeration of the beat-to-beat variability. Adding to the difficulty is the fact that the tracing, which was initiated at a paper speed of 1 cm/minute is switched, at about 11M, for the next 4 minutes to 3 cm/minute. To add to the mischief, the last 16 minutes are recorded at 1 cm/minute. The low amplitude of the uterine contractions and the slow paper speed give the impression of an unusual variant to the uterine contractions. These become less dramatic, less obscure between 11M and 16M, where they are viewed at 3 cm/minute.

This FHR pattern indicates both acute and chronic distress. There are frequent, recurrent, late decelerations, sometimes, but not invariably, combined with variable decelerations with overshoot. Contractions appear about every 3 minutes.

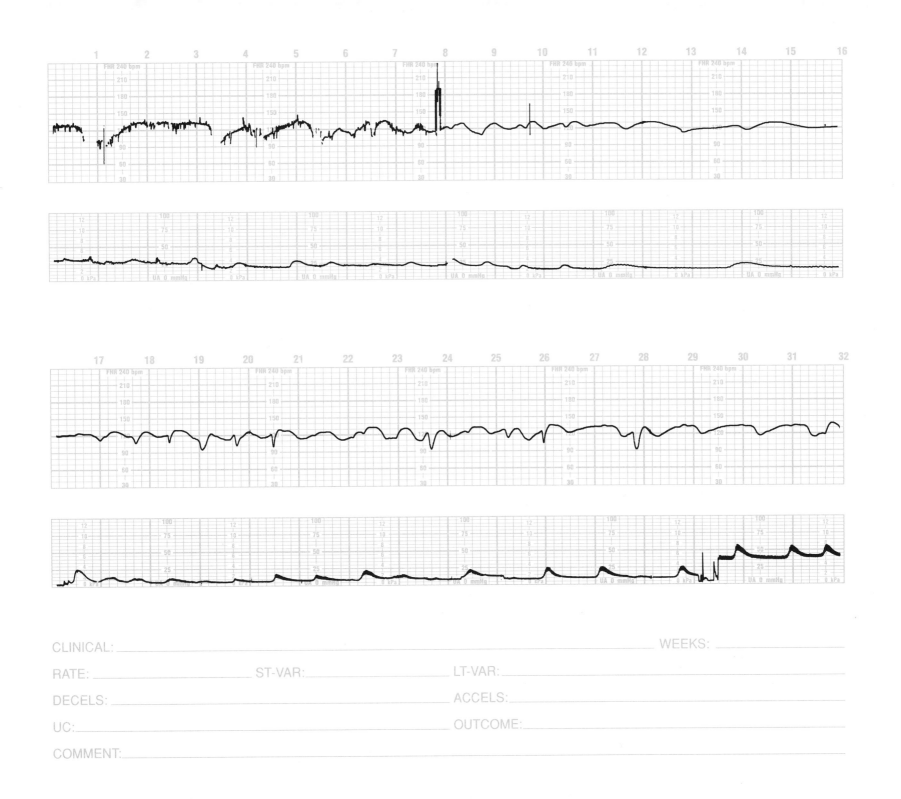

CLINICAL: _____   WEEKS: _____

RATE: _____ ST-VAR: _____   LT-VAR: _____

DECELS: _____   ACCELS: _____

UC: _____   OUTCOME: _____

COMMENT: _____

TRACING: 61

CLINICAL: Oligohydramnios.

WEEKS: 41

BASELINE RATE: 160

STV: Decreased.

LTV: Decreased.

DECELERATIONS: Variable.

ACCELERATIONS: Rebound ("overshoot").

UC: Active labor.

OUTCOME: Neurologic handicap; Apgar scores, 4/6.

COMMENT: This markedly abnormal pattern represents an insult visited on the fetus prior to the onset of monitoring. No comment can be offered on how many weeks or months the pattern has persisted. It is implausible that the pattern was normal 5 or even 15 minutes before the onset of the tracing. Loss of variability to this degree is not a marker of acute, ongoing asphyxia in a previously normal fetus. To reach this point the previously normal fetus will have undergone profound or prolonged asphyxia with recurrent decelerations (late, variable, or prolonged), a rising heart rate, and progressive loss of variability. That sequence would be unlikely to occur in less than 30 minutes but more likely requires an hour or longer. The pattern reveals variable decelerations with overshoot at 2M, 8M, 15M, 20M, 23M, and 31M. When variable decelerations do not overwhelm them, late decelerations appear at 3M (very subtle), 6M, 17M, 23M, and 25M. The asphyxial component, however, produces only a modest drop in the pH to the range of 7.22 to 7.16; the maternal pH is 7.43. The performance of a cesarean section, clearly warranted by the clinical circumstances, may prevent additional insult but is unlikely to result in the birth of a normal infant. See the discussion accompanying tracing 55.

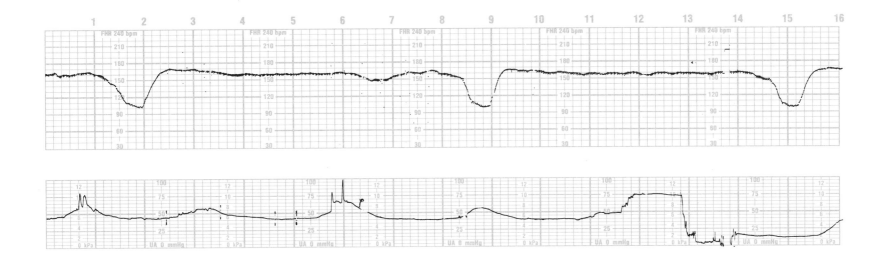

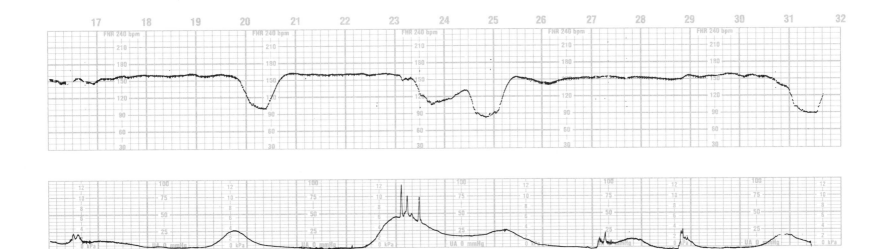

TRACING: 62

CLINICAL: Meconium staining, oligohydramnios.

WEEKS: 41

BASELINE RATE: 140

STV: Absent.

LTV: Absent.

DECELERATIONS: Recurrent variable.

ACCELERATIONS: Rebound ("overshoot").

UC: Late spontaneous labor, pushing with contractions toward end of record.

OUTCOME: Low Apgar scores, dysmature.

COMMENT: This troublesome tracing reveals a stable baseline rate, absent baseline variability, and recurrent variable decelerations with overshoot. The decelerations themselves contain further clues to limited neurologic control over the heart rate. The descending and ascending limbs of the decelerations are relatively leisurely and followed by overshoot. A fetus whose variability is depressed by medication will show variable decelerations with characteristic abrupt changes in the descending slopes and erratic accelerations ("shoulders") following the ascending slopes. The changes seen here are predictable in all respects. The occasional abrupt changes during descent (at 6M and 29M) may represent either arrhythmia or expulsive efforts. Episodes of nodal rhythm appear at the nadir of the deceleration when the rate reaches 60 to 70 bpm (12M, 15M, and 21M). This pattern suggests mild to moderate (but not severe) asphyxia in a chronically compromised fetus. The pattern demands prompt intervention, but neurologic damage may have already taken place.

142

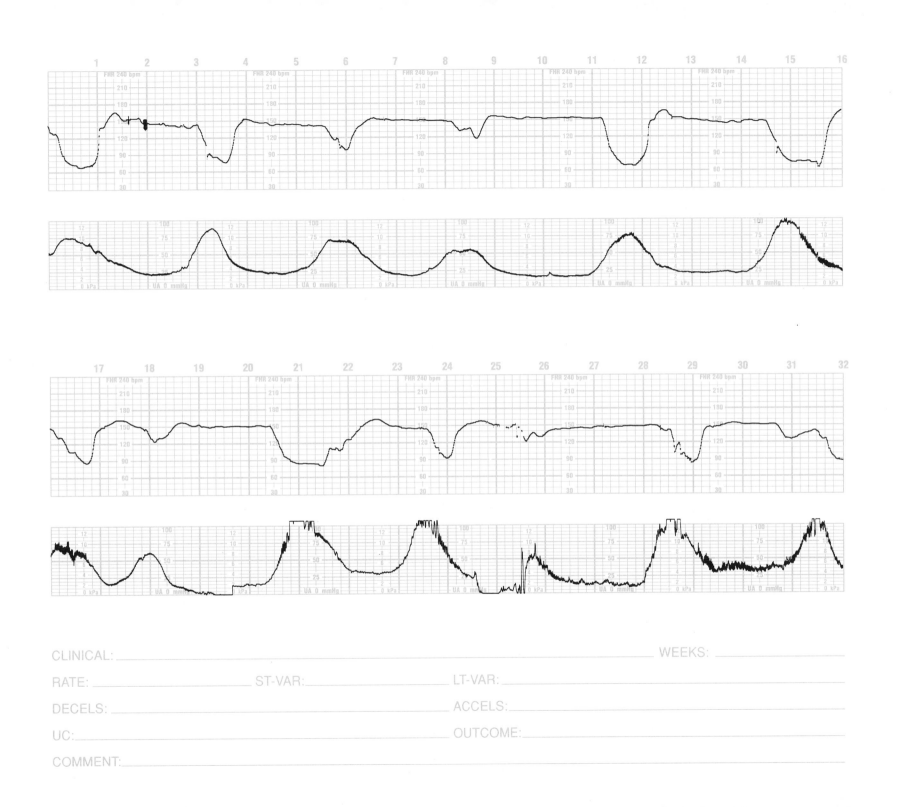

TRACING: 63

CLINICAL: Oligohydramnios.

WEEKS: 41

BASELINE RATE: 150–160

STV: Absent.

LTV: Decreased.

DECELERATIONS: Variable, prolonged.

ACCELERATIONS: Rebound ("overshoot").

UC: Irregular, early labor.

OUTCOME: Apgar scores, 2/4; neurologic handicap.

COMMENT: This chronic pattern reflects long-standing compromise but reveals few decelerations. Note the intermittent "sinusoidal" pattern. Benign sinusoidal patterns usually evolve from, or into, patterns with normal variability. They tend to be more persistent and less regular in their features than those associated with adverse outcomes. Troublesome sinusoidal patterns associated with significant anemia, asphyxia or neurologic handicap reveal persistently absent variability but are otherwise intermittent. Note the absence of spontaneous accelerations. The decelerations at 3M, 15M, and 23M are related to vaginal examination, lateral positioning of the patient, or scalp sampling. Small variable decelerations with overshoot appear at 17M, 19M, and 26M. Scalp sampling reveals the absence of significant fetal asphyxia (scalp pH = 7.31; maternal pH = 7.41). The scalp sampling procedure tends to increase the FHR. For a discussion of the benefits of intervention see tracing 55.

144

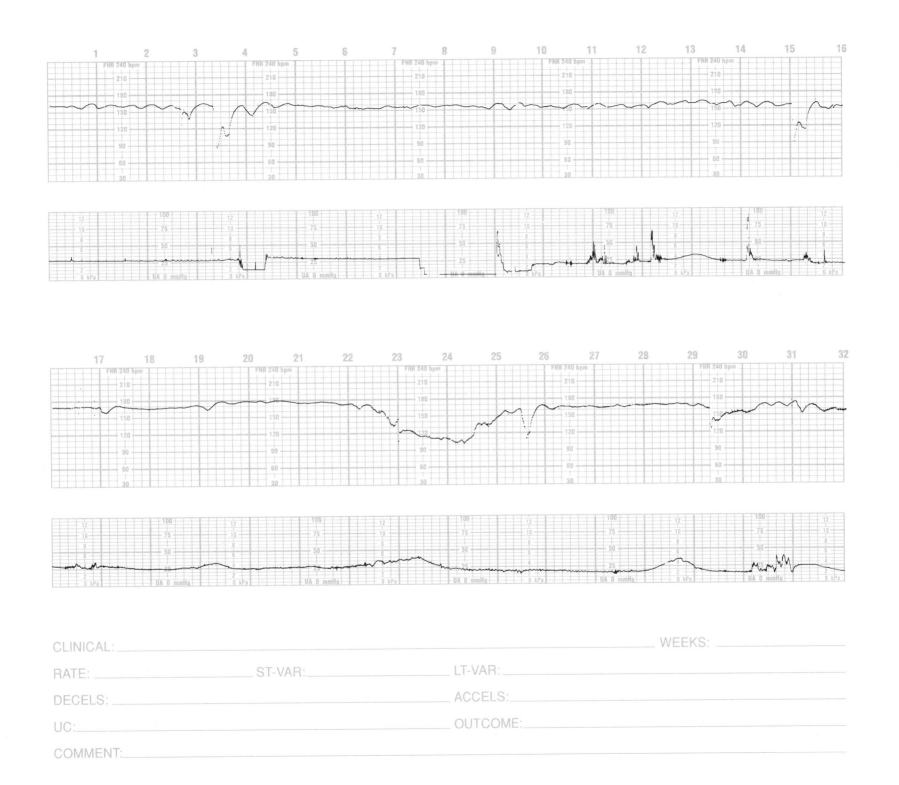

TRACING: 64

CLINICAL: Uneventful pregnancy.

WEEKS: 39

BASELINE RATE: 180

STV: Absent.

LTV: Absent.

DECELERATIONS: Variable, possibly late.

ACCELERATIONS: Rebound ("overshoot").

UC: Infrequent, early labor.

OUTCOME: Apgar scores, 0/0; stillborn.

COMMENT: In this tracing, a continuation of tracing 58, fetal death results from a true knot in the cord. The baseline rate is elevated, long- and short-term baseline variability are absent and small, variable decelerations with overshoot are present. Despite their infrequency, each contraction induces a deceleration that recovers only after 4 to 5 minutes. This may be regarded either as instability of the baseline or a very prolonged, late deceleration. At this point the baby is significantly compromised and intervention is urgently needed. Fetuses with diminished variability on the basis of medication or sleep generally maintain stable baseline rates. If asphyxia develops, decelerations will appear.

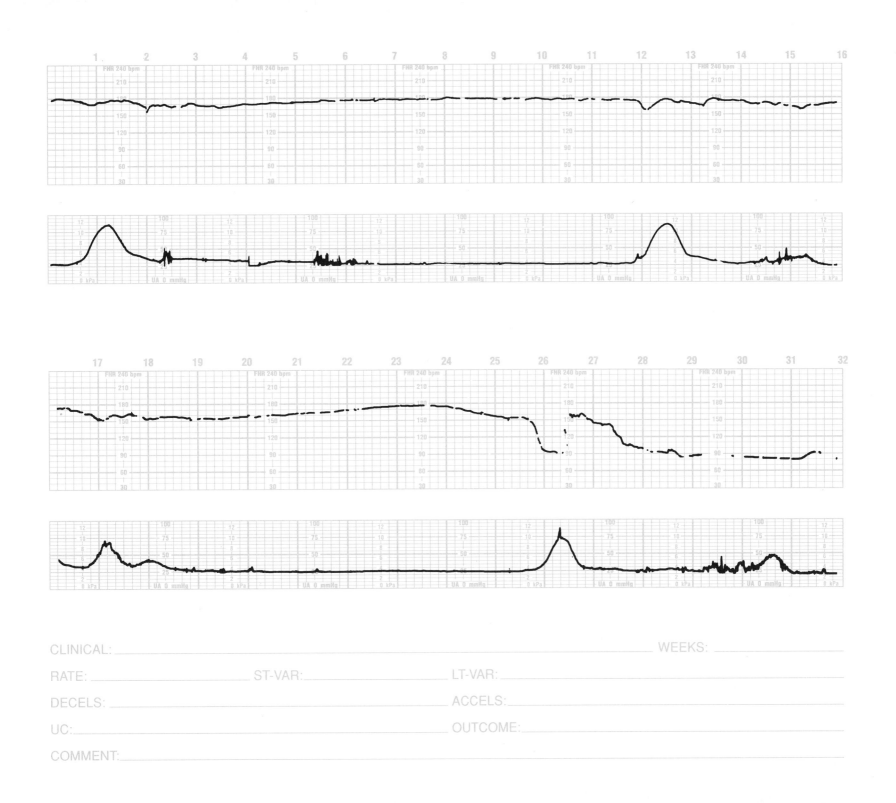

CLINICAL: _____   WEEKS: _____

RATE: _____ ST-VAR: _____   LT-VAR: _____

DECELS: _____   ACCELS: _____

UC: _____   OUTCOME: _____

COMMENT: _____

TRACING: 65

CLINICAL: Preterm labor, uterine anomaly.

WEEKS: 34

BASELINE RATE: 200

STV: Absent.

LTV: Absent.

DECELERATIONS: Variable, undefined.

ACCELERATIONS: Rebound ("overshoot").

UC: Irregular, early labor.

OUTCOME: Apgar scores, 0/0; stillborn.

COMMENT: This tracing illustrates acute deterioration in a chronically affected fetus. Initially, this FHR pattern consists of absent variability, baseline tachycardia, and inconsistent variable decelerations with overshoot. Despite these numerous abnormalities, the first 12 minutes of the tracing are quite stable. Thereafter, the condition of the fetus rapidly (acutely) deteriorates. From then on, the fetus can no longer maintain a stable baseline rate; the baseline falls, the deceleration at 25M evolves into a series of slow oscillations, and the fetus dies.

With this tracing the clinician faces a management decision that will not likely be satisfying. On the one hand, this pattern likely, but not invariably, anticipates subsequent neurologic handicap or death, with little evidence that intervention will change the outcome. In addition, cesarean section imposes some risk to the mother. On the other hand, there is yet enough uncertainty about the outcome during the initial part of the tracing, when it is stable, to consider intervention. At this time, however, there is no evidence that the contractions are exerting any deleterious effect. The last 16 minutes of the tracing are quite hopeless and recovery is quite unlikely.

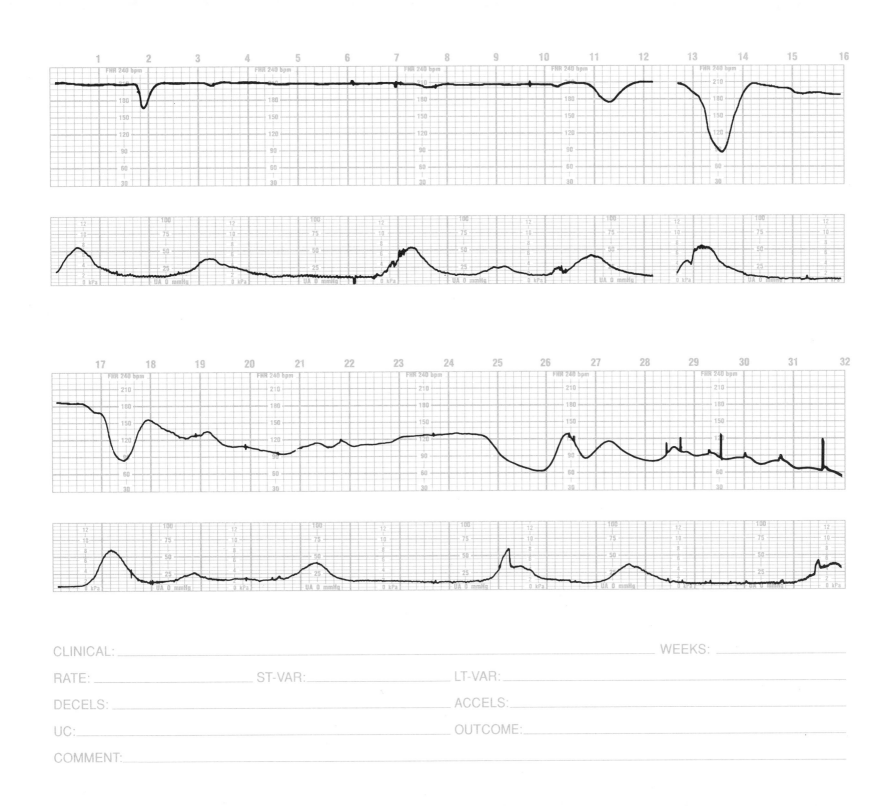

CLINICAL: _____ WEEKS: _____

RATE: _____ ST-VAR: _____ LT-VAR: _____

DECELS: _____ ACCELS: _____

UC: _____ OUTCOME: _____

COMMENT: _____

TRACING: 66

CLINICAL: Abruptio placentae, vaginal bleeding.

WEEKS: 39

BASELINE RATE: Probably 140

STV: Average.

LTV: Average.

DECELERATIONS: Variable, prolonged.

ACCELERATIONS: Exaggerated variable ("shoulders").

UC: Frequent, tachysystole.

OUTCOME: Apgar scores, 0/0; stillborn.

COMMENT: This tracing illustrates recurrent, variable decelerations that deteriorate until fetal death occurs. Notice the rather benign appearance of the initial variable decelerations with the apparent maintenance of baseline variability between the decelerations. Contractions are quite frequent (more often than 1 every 2 minutes). Notice that the recovery phase of the deceleration becomes increasingly more peaked with diminished variability. Immediately after the peaked accelerations, decelerations, probably late, appear. As the condition of the fetus deteriorates, the accelerative peaks become more isolated. Were there more time between contractions, both the baseline rate and the height of the peaks would rise. As this pattern progresses, the variability in the decelerations between the peaks becomes increasingly diminished. Ultimately the baby cannot tolerate this frequency of contractions; the baseline rate falls, decelerations of indefinable character supervene, variability disappears, and the heart rate trails off to fetal death.

This pattern illustrates that variable decelerations do not deteriorate by becoming longer or showing "slow return to the baseline." If anything, the decelerations may become deeper as a result of the rising baseline during the recovery phase, which is not well illustrated here. The inability to retreat to a stable baseline rate and variability, the isolated peaking of the trailing accelerations, and the coalescence into late-appearing decelerations all bespeak deterioration. Finally, the loss of all variability and the inability to maintain a stable heart rate presages terminal bradycardia and death.

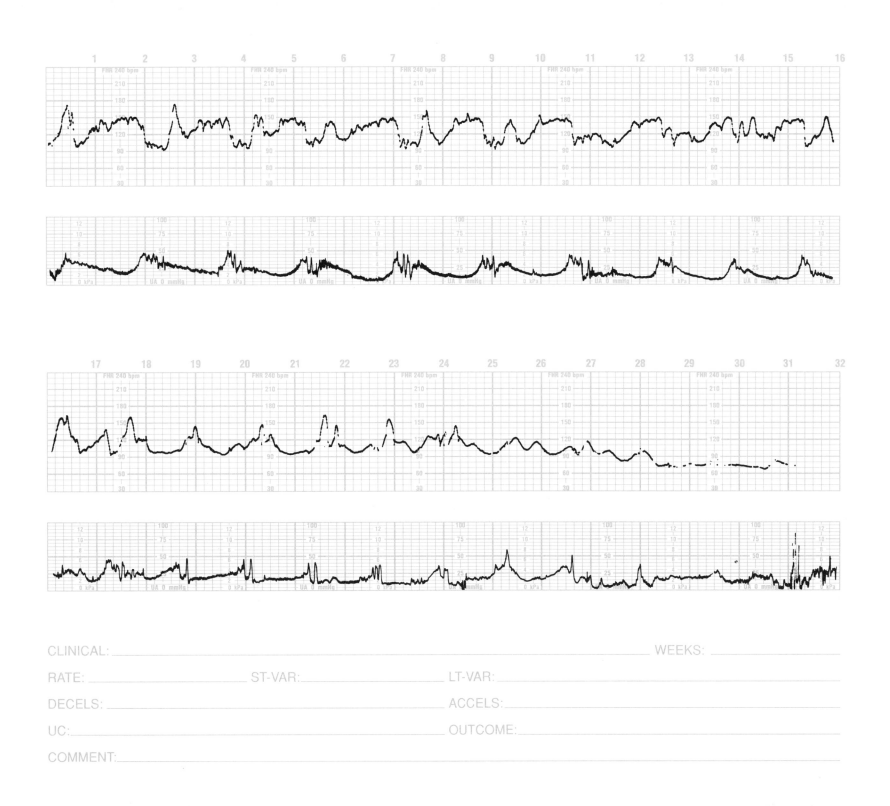

CLINICAL: _____ WEEKS: _____

RATE: _____ ST-VAR: _____ LT-VAR: _____

DECELS: _____ ACCELS: _____

UC: _____ OUTCOME: _____

COMMENT: _____

TRACING: 67

CLINICAL: Pregnancy-induced hypertension.

WEEKS: 38

BASELINE RATE: Not determinable.

STV: Absent.

LTV: Increased.

DECELERATIONS: Variable, prolonged.

ACCELERATIONS: Exaggerated variable ("shoulders").

UC: Hypertonus.

OUTCOME: Apgar scores, 0/0; stillborn.

COMMENT: At the beginning of this tracing the peaked, smoothed accelerations associated with recurrent variable decelerations anticipate fetal deterioration. This pattern is followed (at 14M–16M) by smooth, broad undulations in the heart rate containing some apparent short-term variability (probably artifact). Notice the downward trend of the baseline rate. Uterine contractions of 60 to 70 mm Hg in amplitude and tonus of about 25 mm Hg appear every 3 to 4 minutes. Because of uncertainty about the FHR pattern and the inability to obtain fetal scalp pH, the physician decided upon cesarean section. At the *arrow,* the patient was removed to the delivery room where the monitor was reapplied, revealing an obvious terminal pattern with low heart rate and absent variability. Notice the small accelerations (M20) preceding fetal death. An infant with no respiratory effort or heart rate was delivered 2 minutes later.

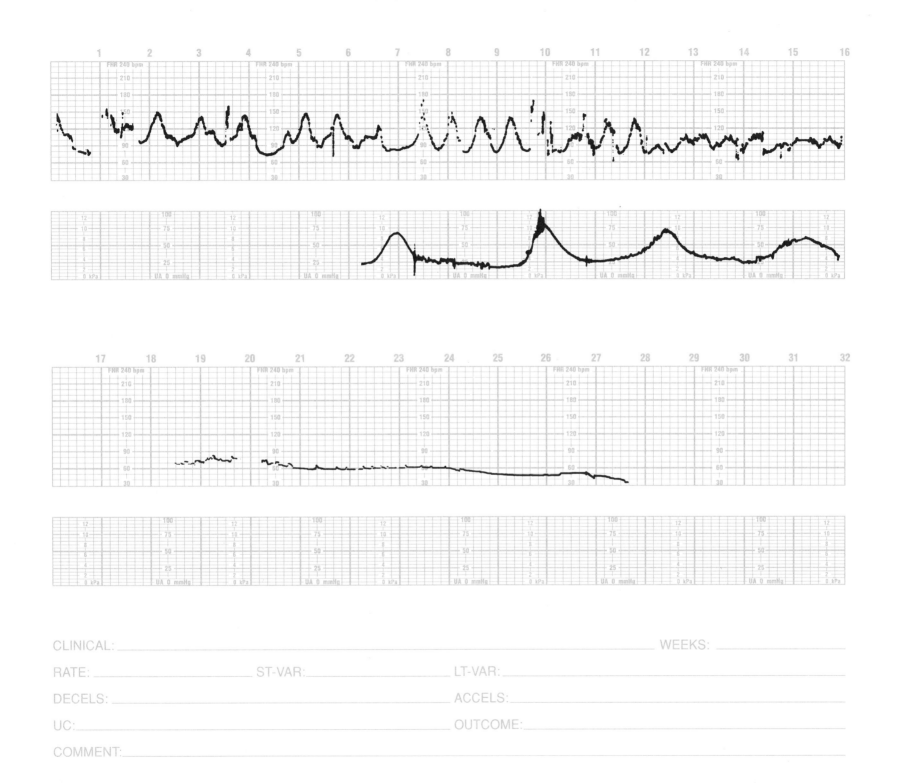

TRACING: 68

CLINICAL: Known hydrocephalic fetus.

WEEKS: 34

BASELINE RATE: 60

STV: Absent.

LTV: Absent.

DECELERATIONS: None.

ACCELERATIONS: Sporadic.

UC: Regular.

OUTCOME: Fetal death.

COMMENT: This tracing illustrates FHR patterns preceding fetal death. The features of baseline bradycardia, absent variability, and undulations in baseline rate, as well as some accelerations in the baseline rate all betray a terminally ill infant. Notice that there are no obvious late decelerations. While every effort should be made to deliver such an infant as rapidly as possible, consistent with maternal safety, it is important to note that by the time the tracing has reached this stage the prospects for survival are bleak at best.

Because the fetus was known to be hydrocephalic and had undergone craniocentesis earlier in labor, no preparations were made for cesarean delivery in this case. The pattern preceding fetal death in anomalous fetuses, however, is usually indistinguishable from those occurring in nonanomalous babies.

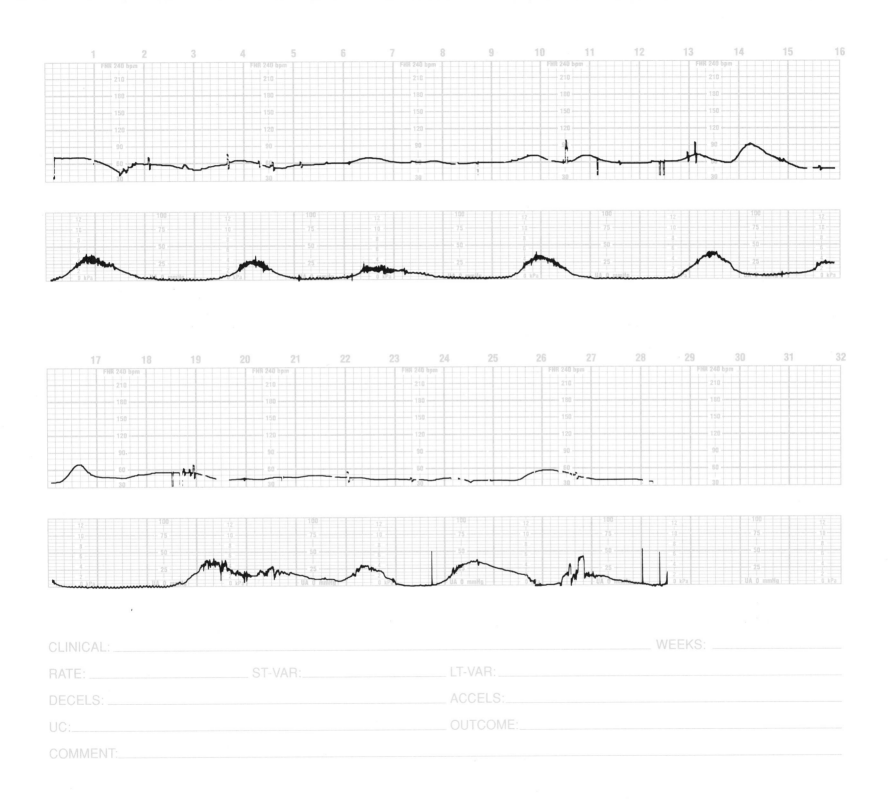

TRACING: 69

CLINICAL: A: Absent fetal movement. B: Maternal lupus erythematosus.

WEEKS: Both: 37

BASELINE RATE: Both: low but not determinable.

STV: Both: Absent.

LTV: A: Average. B: Average, sinusoidal.

DECELERATIONS: A: Probably variable. B: Absent.

ACCELERATIONS: A: Rebound ("overshoot"). B: None.

UC: Both: Frequent, irregular.

OUTCOME: Both: Apgar scores, 0/0; stillborn.

COMMENT: The features of these FHR patterns anticipate the ultimate fetal demise. The baseline rate is in the bradycardic range with absent variability. Small variable decelerations with overshoot punctuate the tracing at 3M, 8M, 9M, and 11M. Other excursions in the rate tend to be predictable undulations rather than true short-term variability. It is impossible to define a baseline heart rate given the frequent contractions and decelerations. The *lower* tracing reveals bradycardia with obvious oscillations, a sinusoidal pattern. Although the correlation of these heart rate patterns with poor outcome and even death is extraordinarily high, it is not yet possible to define heart rate patterns so ominous as to make intervention unnecessary.

156

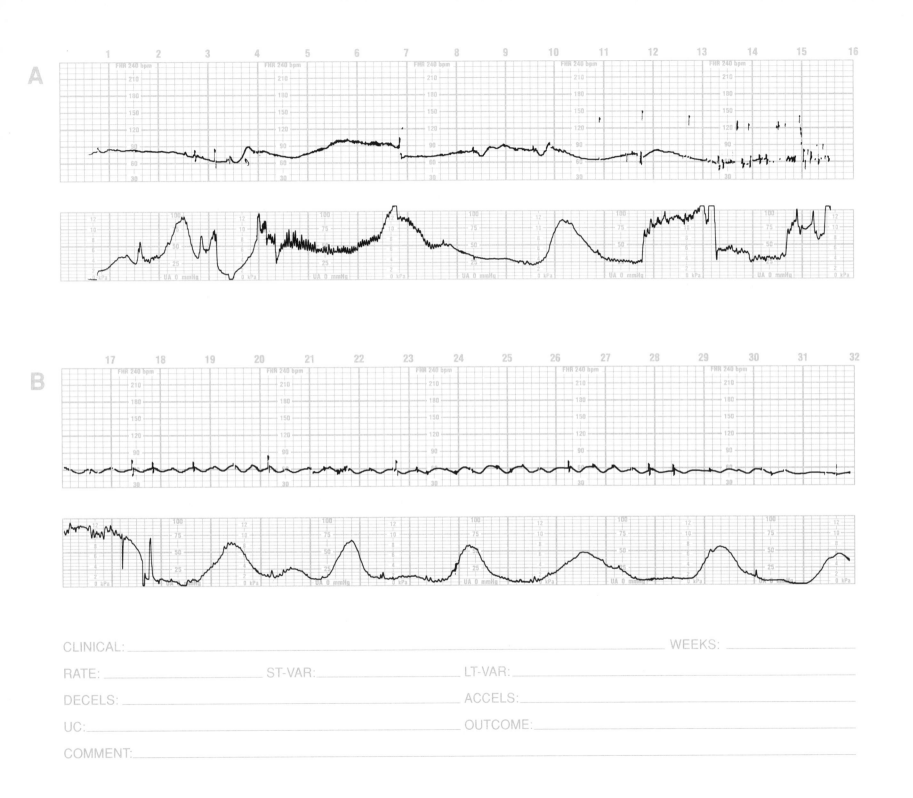

TRACING: 70

CLINICAL: Uneventful prenatal course.

WEEKS: 41

BASELINE RATE: 130

STV: Absent.

LTV: Average to decreased.

DECELERATIONS: Absent.

ACCELERATIONS: Absent.

UC: Oxytocin, tachysystole.

OUTCOME: Apgar scores, 0/0; stillborn; thick meconium.

COMMENT: In this tracing, the absent fetal heart rate variability and intermittent episodes of sinusoidal pattern at 4M, 13M, and 18M augur fetal death. The frequent uterine contractions from excessive oxytocin have no apparent impact on the compromised fetus.

Notice the obvious arrhythmia starting at 23M. This unexpected, 1.5 minute episode of bigeminal heart rate pattern heralds the onset of the bradycardia and fetal death. There are no antecedent episodes of arrhythmia. It has long been suspected that sudden fetal death in utero is related to reflex cardiac arrest of the heart rate. The prevalence of monitoring and the paucity of such cases suggest that if lethal arrhythmias do occur they are essentially terminal events superimposed upon compromised, already asphyxiated fetuses.

A 4,400 g male stillborn infant covered with thick meconium was delivered by cesarean section shortly after this tracing was taken. (Cetrulo CL, Schifrin BS: Fetal heart rate patterns preceding death in utero. *Obstet Gynecol* 1976; 48:521–527.)

158

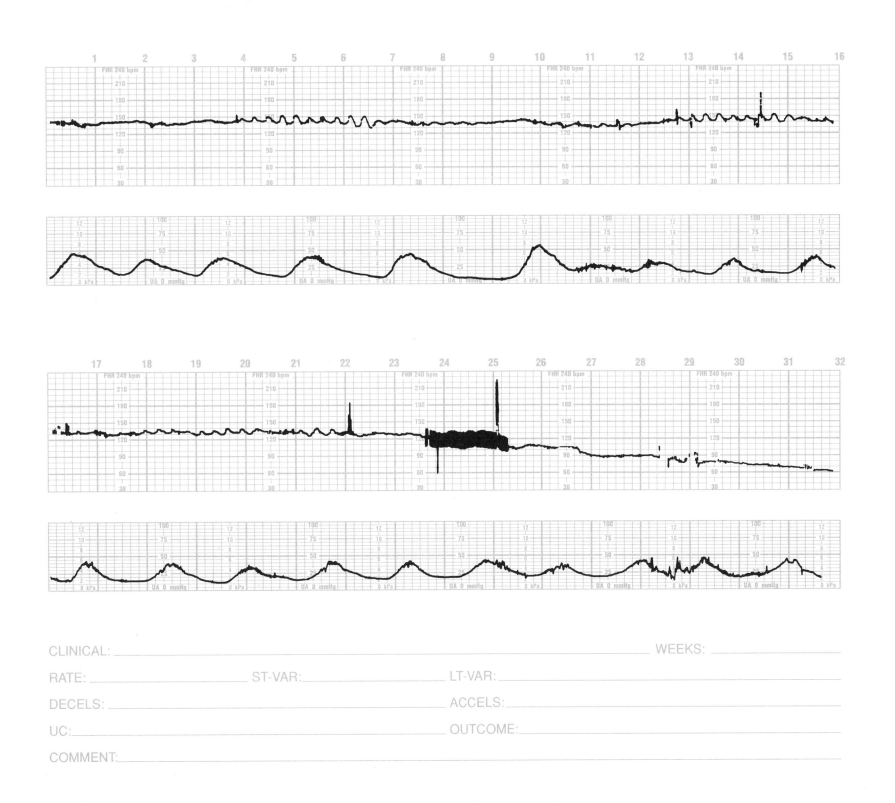

CLINICAL: _____   WEEKS: _____

RATE: _____   ST-VAR: _____   LT-VAR: _____

DECELS: _____   ACCELS: _____

UC: _____   OUTCOME: _____

COMMENT: _____

TRACING: 71

CLINICAL: Irregular fetal heart tones.

WEEKS: 37

BASELINE RATE: 170

STV: Decreased.

LTV: Decreased.

DECELERATIONS: Variable.

ACCELERATIONS: None.

UC: Expulsive efforts, late labor.

OUTCOME: Normal outcome, no evidence of cardiac anomaly. Arrhythmia disappeared within 48 hours.

COMMENT: This tracing reveals fetal arrhythmia—not artifact. While the separation of the two is sometimes difficult, if not impossible, without direct fetal ECG capabilities, there should be no such difficulties with this tracing. Above all, note the recurrent, symmetrical geometric patterns produced by clusters of ectopic beats. Note the suggestion of an arrowhead just after 1M and just before 19M and 28M. This pattern results from cardiac bigeminy (alternating intervals), with the shorter interval getting progressively longer and the longer interval getting progressively shorter. Notice that all of the changes are contained within a narrow range of heart rates (really intervals). These ectopic ventricular beats are multifocal (different heights, different patterns) and frequently alternate with normal beats. For example, with the bigeminy at 25M, there is no line in the middle of the envelope, but there is one in the middle of the run of trigeminy (3M–6M). Notice the occasional decelerations at 7M, 14M, 18M, and 21M. The flat heart rates at 90 bpm between 9M and 10M do not represent decelerations but another form of the arrhythmia. Although the tracing reveals a stable heart rate and probably inconsequential variable decelerations, the frequency of the ectopic beats precludes estimation of the amount of beat-to-beat variability. This tracing mandates ultrasound examination of the fetus to rule out hydrops or congenital anomaly. A scalp sample is unlikely to be helpful. A pediatrician should be present in the delivery room to assist with any resuscitation.

160

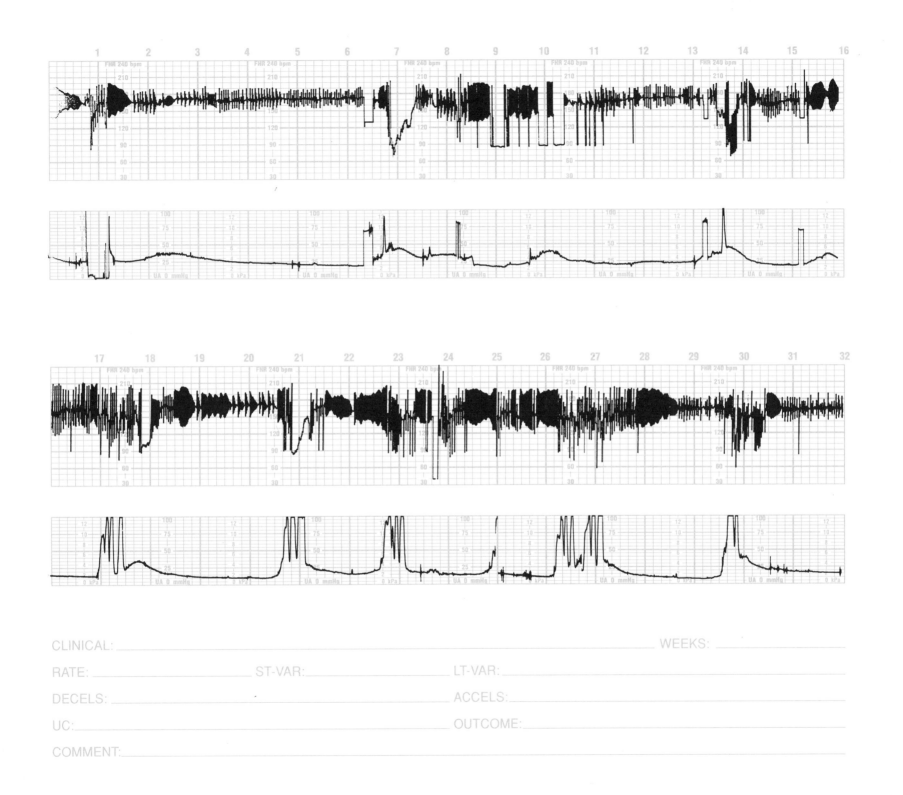

CLINICAL: _____ WEEKS: _____

RATE: _____ ST-VAR: _____ LT-VAR: _____

DECELS: _____ ACCELS: _____

UC: _____ OUTCOME: _____

COMMENT: _____

TRACING: 72

CLINICAL: Uneventful prenatal course.

WEEKS: 38

BASELINE RATE: 150

STV: Average.

LTV: Average.

DECELERATIONS: Variable.

ACCELERATIONS: Sporadic.

UC: Progressing into second stage.

OUTCOME: Apgar scores, 7/9; uneventful neonatal course.

COMMENT: This pattern illustrates variations on the theme of second stage decelerations. As descent begins in this multipara mother, the head of the fetus is high and accelerations dominate the pattern. The vaginal examination between 3M and 4M reveals the cervix to be dilated about 7 cm and induces considerable artifact. Shortly thereafter, variable decelerations appear. The sudden rise in the contraction pressure at 13M suggests a blocked catheter and precludes identification of the true onset of the contraction. Notwithstanding this, the baby demonstrates perfectly satisfactory variability, and in the absence of pushing demonstrates accelerations of the heart rate. Shortly thereafter, variable decelerations begin in earnest as the head comes down the birth canal. After the onset of pushing (24M) we see recurrent decelerations followed by an arrhythmia in its typical location at the end of the deceleration. In contrast to the earlier artifact, these excursions are restrained, limited, create geometric (bigeminal) patterns, and are restricted to the period between contractions. In this situation, the patient should refrain from pushing until the character of the heart rate pattern has defined itself clearly.

162

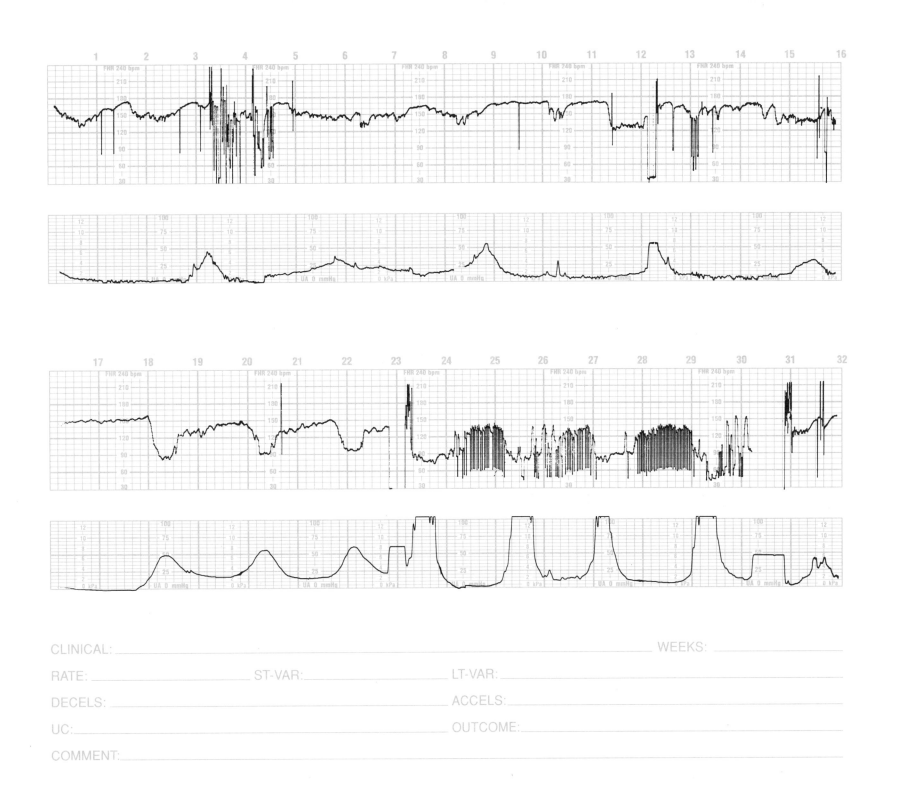

TRACING: 73

CLINICAL: Uneventful pregnancy.

WEEKS: 39

BASELINE RATE: 135

STV: Decreased.

LTV: Decreased.

DECELERATIONS: Absent.

ACCELERATIONS: Absent.

UC: Early labor.

OUTCOME: Apgar scores, 8/9; normal neonatal course.

COMMENT: Conventional wisdom holds that variability is more accurately determined by direct fetal electrode than by external transducers. In this patient, the direct electrode produced a far less interpretable tracing than did the ultrasound transducer. To determine the heart rate and the variability, the monitor must reliably determine each fetal heart beat and then determine the interval between consecutive beats. In this tracing, the calculation of the interval between the regular fetal beats is confounded by the interposition of the large, maternal ECG complex. Normally, the fetal/maternal (signal-to-noise) ratio is about 5:1 or greater. Under such conditions, the detection circuits of the fetal monitor have no difficulty in separating the two and counting only the fetal signal. When the maternal signal is as large as the fetal signal, as in this case, the monitor has considerable difficulty separating the two and counts beats without discrimination. Changing electrodes or monitors will not change this pattern; reverting back to the ultrasound monitor is the most appropriate manuever. Conventional auscultation will also reveal the regular fetal heart rate.

164

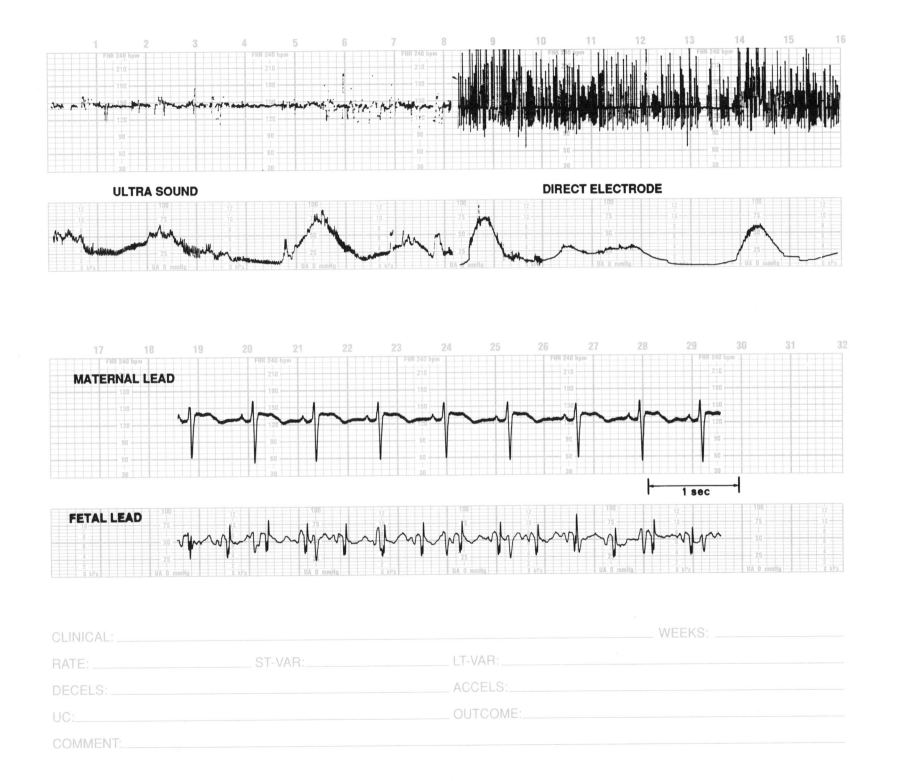

ULTRA SOUND

DIRECT ELECTRODE

MATERNAL LEAD

1 sec

FETAL LEAD

CLINICAL: _____   WEEKS: _____

RATE: _____   ST-VAR: _____   LT-VAR: _____

DECELS: _____   ACCELS: _____

UC: _____   OUTCOME: _____

COMMENT: _____

TRACING: 74

CLINICAL: Maternal fever, nuchal cord.

WEEKS: 39

BASELINE RATE: 190–200

STV: Diminished to average.

LTV: Decreased.

DECELERATIONS: Late, variable, prolonged.

ACCELERATIONS: None.

UC: Exuberant response to oxytocin yielding tachysystole.

OUTCOME: Apgar scores, 7/8; emergency low forceps delivery.

COMMENT: This tracing illustrates the impact of artifact in the heart rate channel on the evaluation of baseline variability and the impact of excessive maternal movement on the evaluation of uterine activity. Superficially, the abrupt, limited vertical lines ("picket fence") that dominate the upper tracing may represent arrhythmia or artifact. The decision that it is artifact is made by close observation of the sequence of the excursions. In some of the spikes, the initial deflection is upward while in the others, the initial deflection is downward. Arrhythmia would tend to produce similar deflections in all complexes. The flat lines in both channels between 22M and 24M also represent artifact—a result of the patient having been disconnected from the monitor. The monitor has been turned off at 23M. When the monitor is restarted, the UC recording increases in intensity as the heat of the pen stylus increases. (This is an early-generation Corometrics monitor.) The exaggerated, chaotic deflections between 25M and 26M+ are artifact.

The elevated baseline rate and diminished variability (where it can be determined) are the result of the fever. The development of late decelerations followed by rising baseline at 10M and thereafter represents transient acute fetal distress related to the excessive frequency of uterine contractions induced by oxytocin. Recovery has already begun by 11M when the contraction frequency has diminished and late decelerations are no longer present. Following 16M there is a break in the record of 8 minutes. By 17M, recovery from the initial insult is nearly complete. But as the fetus descends, variable decelerations become apparent and the patient is moved to the delivery room. There the fetus appears to have recovered (24M+), but a prolonged deceleration supervenes, associated with relentless pushing. The baby is delivered by an emergency low forceps procedure at the end of the tracing.

Proper functioning of the tocotransducer is required for proper evaluation of uterine contractions. If excessive maternal movement or obesity interferes with proper registration of contractions, then an internal catheter should be inserted if possible.

166

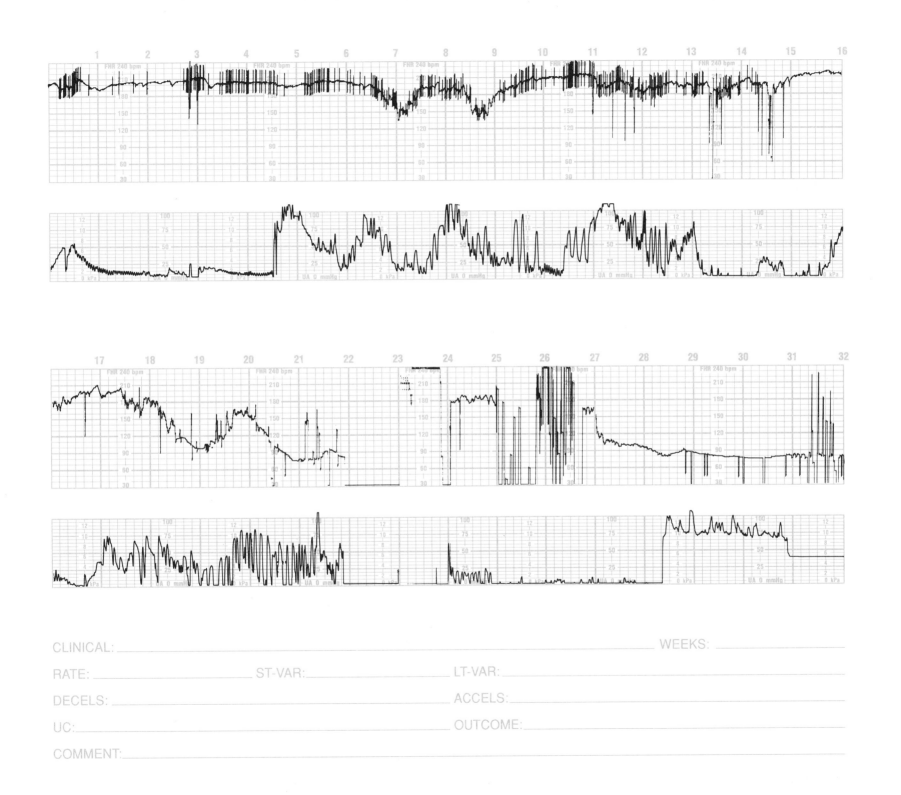

CLINICAL: _____   WEEKS: _____

RATE: _____   ST-VAR: _____   LT-VAR: _____

DECELS: _____   ACCELS: _____

UC: _____   OUTCOME: _____

COMMENT: _____

TRACING: 75

CLINICAL: Any guess.

WEEKS: Pick one.

BASELINE RATE: Your choice.

STV: Absent, decreased, average, increased.

LTV: Same.

DECELERATIONS: Variable (no lates!).

ACCELERATIONS: Numerous.

UC: Early active labor.

OUTCOME: One not so good.

COMMENT: This mischievous tracing illustrates both the range of variability as well as the uniqueness of individual heart rate patterns. As a single tracing, the abrupt changes in the baseline heart rate and variability at 9M, 16M, and 25M are physiologically implausible. Indeed, these panels represent the tracings of four different fetuses of four different mothers. While there will be some fluctuation in the amount of variability during labor, the individual fetus attempts to maintain a stable baseline rate. As a result of stress, medication, maternal provocation, or change in fetal state, the baseline rate may rise but it does so only slowly—never instantaneously. The only exception to this rule is an arrhythmia, which may produce an abrupt, instantaneous rise or fall in the rate. If you find abrupt change of pattern in a tracing consider either (1) a second fetus or (2) the mother as the probable source. None of the patterns here reveals fetal distress.

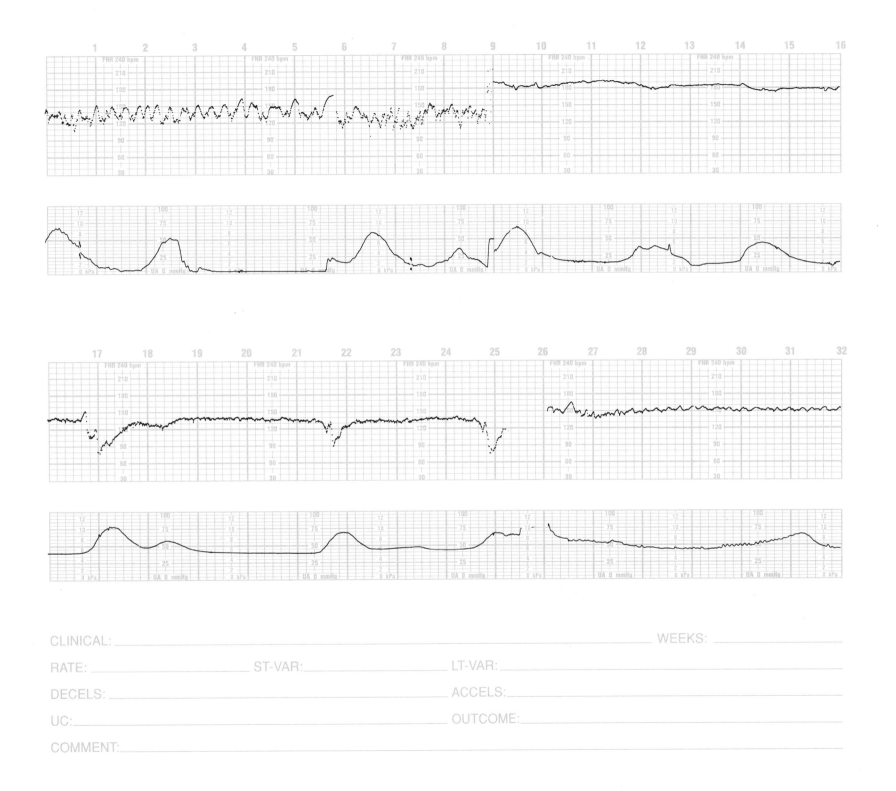

TRACING: 76

CLINICAL: Polyhydramnios.

WEEKS: 34

BASELINE RATE: 200/130

STV: Absent.

LTV: Diminished.

DECELERATIONS: Variable.

ACCELERATIONS: Rebound ("overshoot"), unclassified (30M).

UC: Late labor.

OUTCOME: Multiple congenital anomalies incompatible with life.

COMMENT: This tracing and the following one (tracing 77), both derived from the same fetus, are offered here to startle and puzzle the reader. Even superficial inspection will reveal that the tracing is most abnormal. But is the baby asphyxiated? The tracing begins with a flat heart rate at 200 bpm, accompanied by usually small, variable decelerations with overshoot at 3M, 6M+, 13M, and 14M. At 17M we find an abrupt descent to a stable rate of 140 bpm with equally diminished variability. From this new rate, usually small, variable decelerations with overshoot appear at 19M, 21M, and 25M. The overshoot after 25M defies description. It presents with an abrupt, angular upswing at 25M+ and a sudden transient downswing just after 26M. The same problem arises in the description of the acceleration at 30M. The gradual rise is followed by an acute, right-angle deflection upward, a slow decay, and a right-angle deflection downward. Thus we have two separate heart rates, each stable, each giving off both abnormal or bizarre accelerations and decelerations. The tracing continues on the next panel.

170

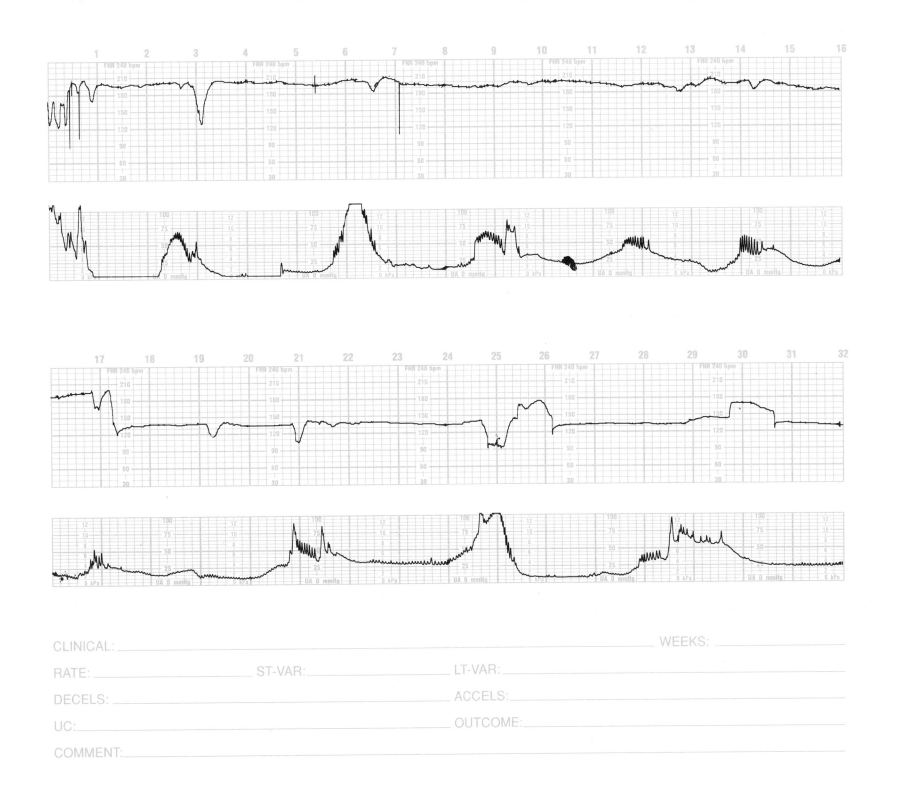

TRACING: 77

CLINICAL: Polyhydramnios.

WEEKS: 34

BASELINE RATE: 180/130

STV: Absent.

LTV: Diminished.

DECELERATIONS: Variable.

ACCELERATIONS: Rebound ("overshoot").

UC: Late labor.

OUTCOME: Multiple congenital anomalies incompatible with life.

COMMENT: This pattern continues from the previous tracing (tracing 76). From a baseline of about 130 bpm the heart rate decelerates for about 1 minute and then, with fits and starts, returns over the next 5 minutes to the earlier baseline rate and variability. At 11M we find a variable deceleration whose amplitude exceeds 100 bpm, lasting 1 minute, that does not recur despite significant pushing with contractions. Indeed, subsequent contractions are much more likely to be associated with accelerations (really variable decelerations with overshoot) than decelerations.

Just as this sequence does not represent normal responsiveness, neither does it represent asphyxia. The presence of accelerations, the absence of repetitive decelerations, and the maintenance of a stable baseline rate all contraindicate asphyxia. The abnormalities in the tracing are unique and do not fit any normal definition of accelerations.

This fetus has multiple congenital anomalies involving both the heart and the central nervous system. The more bizarre the pattern and the more "mixed signals" it gives off, the more one should consider congenital anomaly in the differential diagnosis.

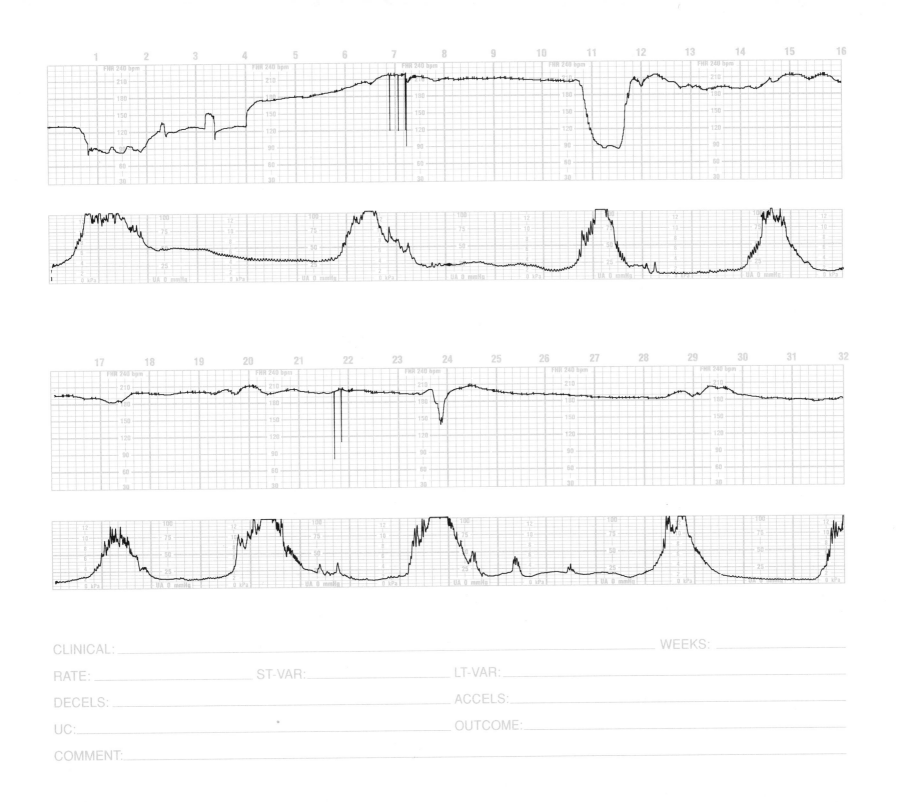

TRACING: 78

CLINICAL: Hydranencephalic fetus.

WEEKS: 34

BASELINE RATE: Depends upon epoch.

STV: Pick one.

LTV: Absent.

DECELERATIONS: Prolonged, late.

ACCELERATIONS: Abnormal, peaked.

UC: Regular.

OUTCOME: Apgar scores, 0/0; stillborn; hydranencephaly.

COMMENT: These tracings illustrate three epochs preceding death in an anomalous fetus. In *panel A* exaggerated beat-to-beat variability accompanies unique, peaked, isolated accelerations. Neither the accelerations nor the variability is normal or reassuring. Normal accelerations tend to be broader, less peaked, and less symmetrical. Normal variability tends to show both long- and short-term features and to be much less predictable than the high-frequency, low-amplitude changes seen here.

Panel B, obtained after the removal of 900 cc of cerebrospinal fluid, suggests an elevated baseline without variability; defining the baseline is difficult as the fetus is either entering or recovering from a deceleration. Each prolonged deceleration returns only slowly to the baseline—so-called late recovery. When decelerations recover slowly to a high baseline with decreased variability they may reasonably be regarded as ominous. "Slow return" to a previous normal baseline with maintenance of variability suggests no adverse context. The "sawtooth" excursions during the recovery phase of the decelerations may represent injury to primitive areas of the brain. They are occasionally seen in profoundly asphyxiated fetuses in whom intracranial hemorrhage later develops. *Panel C* represents the terminal episode with marked bradycardia, recurrent late decelerations, and fetal death.

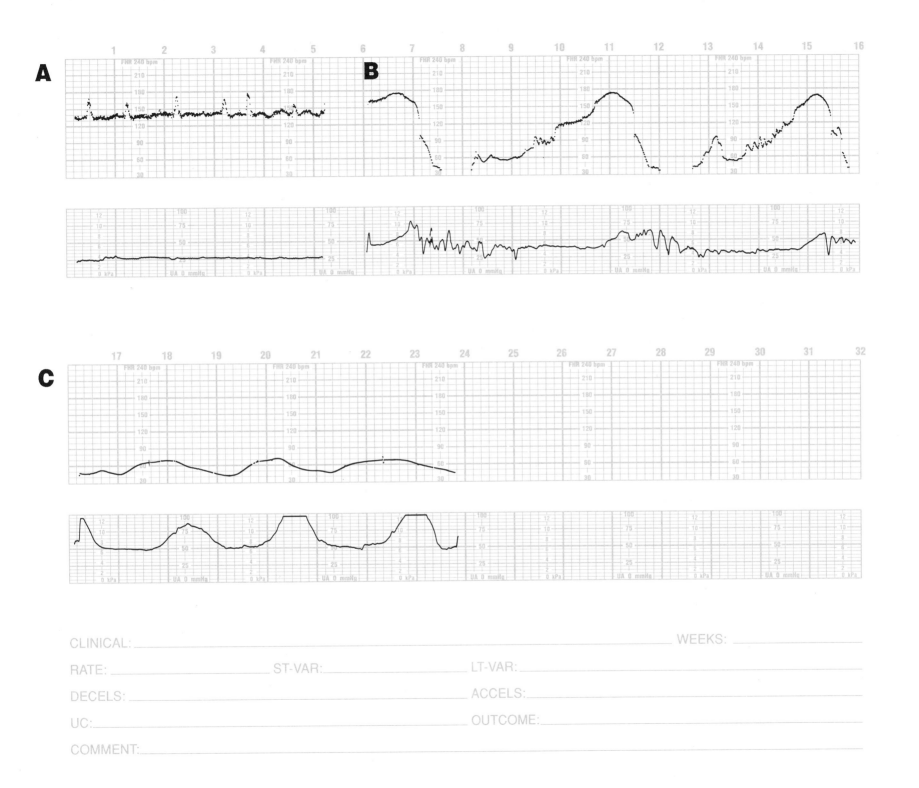

REFERENCES

Adams RD, Prod'hom LS, Rabinowicz TH: Intrauterine brain death. *Acta Neuropathol* 1977; 40:41.

Adamsons K, Beard RW, Myers RE: Comparison of the composition of arterial venous and capillary blood of the fetal monkey during labor. *Am J Obstet Gynecol* 1970; 107:435–440.

Adamson K, Myers RE: Late decelerations and brain tolerance of the fetal monkey to intrapartum asphyxia. *Am J Obstet Gynecol* 1977; 128:893.

Afriat C, Schifrin BS: Sources of error in fetal heart rate monitoring. *J Obstet Gynecol Neonat Nurs* 1976; 12:11–15.

Aladjem S, Feria A, Rest J, et al: Fetal heart rate responses to fetal movements. *Br J Obstet Gynaecol* 1977; 84:487–491.

Amato J: Fetal monitoring in a community hospital. *Obstet Gynecol* 1977; 50:269–274.

Arias F: Intrauterine resuscitation with terbutaline: A method for the management of acute intrapartum fetal distress. *Am J Obstet Gynecol* 1978; 131:39.

Barcroft J: *Researches on Prenatal Life.* Springfield, Ill, Charles C Thomas Publisher, 1947.

Barham KA: Amnioscopy, meconium, and fetal well-being. *J Obstet Gynaecol Br Comm* 1969; 76:412.

Baskett TF, Koh KS: Sinusoidal fetal heart rate pattern: A sign of fetal hypoxia. *Obstet Gynecol* 1974; 44:379.

Benson RC, Shubeck F, Deutschberger J, et al: Fetal heart rate as a predictor of fetal distress. A report from the collaborative project. *Obstet Gynecol* 1968; 32:259–266.

Boehm FH: Prolonged end stage fetal heart rate deceleration. *Obstet Gynecol* 1975; 45:579–582.

Boehm FH: FHR variability, key to fetal well-being. *Contemp Obstet Gynecol* 1977; 9:57–65.

Boehm F, Growdon J: The effect of eclamptic convulsions on the fetal heart rate. *Am J Obstet Gynecol* 1974; 120:851–852.

Bowe ET, Beard RW, Finster M, et al: Reliability of fetal blood sampling, maternal-fetal relationships. *Am J Obstet Gynecol* 1970; 107:279–287.

Brann AW, Myers RE: Central nervous system findings in the newborn monkey following severe in utero partial asphyxia. *Neurology* 1975; 25:327–338.

Bronatek V, Scheffs J: The pathogenesis and significance of saltatory patterns in the fetal heart rate. *Int J Gynaecol Obstet* 1973; 11:223.

Bruce SL, James LS, Bowe ET, et al: Umbilical cord complication as a cause of perinatal morbidity and mortality. *J Perinat Med* 1978; 6:89.

Cabal LA, Siassi B, Zanini B, et al: Factors affecting heart rate variability in preterm infants. *Pediatrics* 1980; 65:50.

Caldeyro-Barcia, Mendez-Bauer C, Poseiro JJ, et al: Control of human fetal heart rate during labor, in Cassels DE (ed): *The Heart and circulation in the Newborn and Infant.* New York, Grune & Stratton, 1966, pp 7–36.

Carson BS, Losey RW, Bowes WA, et al: Combined obstetric and pediatric approach to prevent meconium aspiration syndrome. *Am J Obstet Gynecol* 1976; 126:712.

Cetrulo CL, Schifrin BS: Fetal heart rate patterns preceding death in utero. *Obstet Gynecol* 1976; 48:521–527.

Cibils LA: Clinical significance of fetal heart rate patterns during labor: Variable decelerations. *Am J Obstet Gynecol* 1975; 132:791–805.

Cohen WR, Schifrin BS: Diagnosis and treatment of fetal distress, in Bolognese RJ, Schwarz RH, Schneider J (eds): *Perinatal Medicine*, ed 2. Baltimore, Williams & Wilkins, 1982, pp 223–243.

Cohen WR, Schifrin BS, Doctor G: Elevation of the fetal presenting part: A method of intrauterine resuscitation. *Am J Obstet Gynecol* 1975; 123:646.

Cohn HE, Piasecki GJ, Jackson BT: Effect of atropine blockade on the fetal cardiovascular response to hypoxemia. *Gynecol Invest* 1976; 7:57.

Cohn HE, Piasecki GJ, Jackson BJ: The effect of fetal heart rate on cardiovascular function during hypoxemia. *Am J Obstet Gynecol* 1980; 138:1190.

Cohn HE, Sacks EJ, Heymann MA, et al: Cardiovascular responses to hypoxemia and acidemia in fetal lambs. *Am J Obstet Gynecol* 1974; 120:817.

Comline RS, Silver M: Development of activity in the adrenal medulla of the foetus and new-born animal. *Br Med Bull* 1966; 22:16.

Cordero L Jr, Hon EG: Scalp abscess: A rare complication of fetal monitoring. *J Pediatr* 1971; 78:533–536.

Dalton KJ, Phil D, Dawes GS, et al: The autonomic nervous system and fetal heart rate variability. *Am J Obstet Gynecol* 1983; 146:456.

Dawes G: *Foetal and Neonatal Physiology.* Chicago, Year Book Medical Publishers, 1968.

Dawes GS, Gardner WN, Johnston BM, et al: Breathing in fetal lambs: The effects of brain stem section. *J Physiol* 1983; 335:535.

Day E, Maddern C, Wood C: Auscultation of foetal heart rate: An assessment of its error and significance. *Br Med J* 1968; 4:422–424.

de Haan J, van Bemmel JH, Stolte LAM, et al: Quantitative evaluation of the fixed heart rate during pregnancy and labor. *Eur J Obstet Gynecol* 1971; 3:103.

De Souza SW, Richards B: Neurological sequelae in newborn babies after perinatal asphyxia. *Arch Dis Child* 1978; 53:564–569.

Divon MY, Muskat Y, Platt LD, et al: Increased beat-to-beat variability during uterine contractions: A common association in uncomplicated labor. *Am J Obstet Gynecol* 1984; 149:893–896.

Divon MY, Yeh SY, Zimmer EZ, et al: Respiratory sinus arrhythmia in the human fetus. *Am J Obstet Gynecol* 1985; 151:425–428.

Erkolla R, Gronroos M, Punnonen R, et al: Analysis of intrapartum fetal deaths: Their decline with increasing electronic fetal monitoring. *Acta Obstet Gynecol Scand* 1984;63:459–462.

Fenton AN, Steer CM: Fetal distress. *Am J Obstet Gynecol* 1962; 83:354.

Fernandez-Rocha L, Oulette R: Fetal bleeding: An unusual complication of fetal monitoring. *Am J Obstet Gynecol* 1976; 125:1153–1155.

Fleischer A, Schulman H, Jagani N, et al: The development of fetal acidosis in the presence of an abnormal fetal heart rate tracing: I. The average for gestational age fetus. *Am J Obstet Gynecol* 1982; 144:55.

Freeman RK, Schifrin BS: Whither paracervical block? *Int Anesth Clin* 1973; 11:69–91.

Freeman RK, James J: Clinical experience with the oxytocin challenge test: II. An ominous atypical pattern. *Obstet Gynecol* 1977; 46:255.

Gabbe S, Ettinger B, Freeman R, et al: Umbilical cord compression associated with amniotomy: Laboratory observations. *Am J Obstet Gynecol* 1976; 126:353–355.

Gal D, Jacobson LM, Ser H, et al: Sinusoidal pattern: An alarming sign of fetal distress. *Am J Obstet Gynecol* 1978; 132:903.

Garite TJ, Linzey EM, Freeman RK, et al: Fetal heart rate patterns and fetal distress in fetuses with congenital anomalies. *Obstet Gynecol* 1979; 53:716–720.

Gaziano EP: A study of variable decelerations in association with other heart rate patterns during monitored labor. *Am J Obstet Gynecol* 1979; 135:360–363.

Gibbs RS, Jones PM, Wilder CJY: Internal fetal monitoring and maternal infection following cesarean section: A prospective study. *Obstet Gynecol* 1978; 53:193–197.

Gleicher N, Runowicz CD, Brown BL: Sinusoidal fetal heart rate pattern in association with amnionitis. *Obstet Gynecol* 1980; 56:109–111.

Glick G, Braunwald E: Relative roles of the sympathetic and parasympathetic nervous systems in the control of heart rate. *Circ Res* 1965; 16:363.

Goodlin RC, Lowe EW: A functional umbilical cord occlusion heart rate pattern: The significance of overshoot. *Obstet Gynecol* 1974; 43:22.

Goodlin RC, Schmidt W: Human fetal arousal levels as indicated by heart rate recordings. *Am J Obstet Gynecol* 1972; 114:613.

Gray JH, Cudmore DW, Luther ER, et al: Sinusoidal fetal heart rate pattern associated with alphaprodine administration. *Obstet Gynecol* 1978; 52:678–681.

Green JN, Paul RH: The value of amniocentesis in prolonged pregnancy. *Obstet Gynecol* 1978; 51:293.

Gregory GA, Gooding CA, Phibbs RH, et al: Meconium aspiration in infants—a prospective study. *J Pediatr* 1974; 85:848.

Greiss FCH: Concepts of uterine blood flow, in Wynn R (ed): *Obstetrics and Gynecology Annual*. New York, Appleton-Century Crofts, 1973, p 55.

Greiss FC, Still GJ, Anderson SG: Effects of local anesthetic agents on the uterine vasculatures and myometrium. *Am J Obstet Gynecol* 1976; 124:889.

Greenfield ADM, Shepherd JT: Cardiovascular responses to asphyxia on the foetal guinea pig. *Physiology* 1953; 120:538.

Griffin RL, Caron FJM, van Geijn HP: Behavioral states in the human fetus during labor. *Am J Obstet Gynecol* 1985; 152:828–833.

Hagberg B, Hagberg G, Olow I: The changing panorama of cerebral palsy in Sweden 1954–70. *Acta Paediatr Scand* 1975; 64:187–200.

Hammacher K: The clinical significance of cardiotocography, in Huntingford PS, Huter EA, Saling E (eds): *Perinatal Medicine*. Georg Thieme Verlag, KG, Stuttgart, 1969, pp 80–93.

Hammacher K, Huter KA, Bokelmann J, et al: Foetal heart frequency and condition of the foetus and newborn. *Gynecologia* 1968; 166:349.

Harris JL, Krueger TR, Parer JT: Mechanisms of late decelerations of the fetal heart rate during hypoxia. *Am J Obstet Gynecol* 1982; 144:491.

Haverkamp AD, et al: A controlled trial of the differential effect of intrapartum monitoring. *Am J Obstet Gynecol* 1979; 134:399.

Herbert CM, Boehm FH: Prolonged end-stage fetal heart rate deceleration: A reanalysis. *Obstet Gynecol* 1981; 57:589–593.

Hobbins JC, Grannum PAT, Romero R, et al: Percutaneous umbilical blood sampling. *Am J Obstet Gynecol* 1985; 152:1–6.

Hon EH, Quilligan EJ: The classification of fetal heart rate: II. A revised working classification. *Conn Med* 1967; 31:779.

Hon EH, Khazin AF, Paul RH: Biochemical studies of the fetus: II. Fetal pH and Apgar scores. *Obstet Gynecol* 1969; 33:237–255.

Hon EH, Bradfield AH, Hess OW: The electronic evaluation of the fetal heart rate: V. The vagal factor in fetal bradycardia. *Am J Obstet Gynecol* 1961; 82:291.

Humphrey MD, Chang A, Wood EC: A decrease in fetal pH during the second stage of labor when conducted in the dorsal position. *Br J Obstet Gynaecol* 1974; 81:600–602.

Hutson JM, Mueller-Heubach E: Diagnosis and management of intrapartum reflex fetal heart rate changes. *Clin Perinatol* 1982; 9:325.

Ibarra-Polo AA, Guiloff FE, Gomez-Rogers C: Fetal heart rate throughout pregnancy. *Am J Obstet Gynecol* 113:814–818.

Ingemarsson E, Ingemarsson I, Svenningsen NW: Impact of routine fetal monitoring during labour on fetal outcome with long-term follow-up. *Am J Obstet Gynecol* 1974; 141:529.

Itskovitz J, LaGamma EF, Rudolph AM: Heart rate and blood pressure responses to umbilical cord compression in fetal lambs with special reference to the mechanism of variable deceleration. *Am J Obstet Gynecol* 1983; 147:451.

Iwamoto HS, Rudolph AM, Keil LC, et al: Hemodynamic responses of the sheep fetus to vasopressin infusion. *Circ Res* 1979; 44:430.

Jacobson L, Rooth G: Interpretative aspects of the acid base composition and its variation in fetal scalp blood and maternal blood during labor. *Br J Obstet Gynaecol* 1971; 78:971.

James LS, Yeh MN, Morishima HO, et al: Umbilical vein occlusion and transient acceleration of the fetal heart rate. *Am J Obstet Gynecol* 1976; 126:276.

Johnson TRB, Compton AA, Rotmensch J, et al: Significance of the sinusoidal fetal heart rate pattern. *Am J Obstet Gynecol* 1981; 139:446–453.

Kariniemi V, Lehtovirta P, Rauramo I, et al: Effects of smoking on fetal heart rate variability during gestational weeks 27 to 32. *Am J Obstet Gynecol* 1984; 149:575–576.

Kates RB, Schifrin BS: Fetal cardiac asystole during labor. *Obstet Gynecol* 1986; 67:549–555.

Keegan K, Waffarn F, Quilligan E: Obstetric characteristics and fetal heart rate patterns of infants who convulse during the newborn period. *Am J Obstet Gynecol* 1985; 153:732.

Kelso IM, Parson RJ, Lawrence GF, et al: An assessment of continuous fetal heart rate monitoring in labor. *Am J Obstet Gynecol* 1978; 131:526–532.

Kero P, Antila K, Ylitalo V, et al: Decreased heart rate variation in decerebration syndrome: Quantitative clinical criterion of brain death? *Pediatrics* 1978; 62:307.

Knuppel RA, Cetrulo CL: Fetal acidosis and a low Apgar in the presence of meconium staining and a normal fetal heart rate pattern: A case report. *J Reprod Med* 1978; 21:241.

Krebs HB, Petres RE, Dunn LJ, et al: Intrapartum fetal heart rate monitoring: I. Classification and prognosis of fetal heart rate patterns. *Am J Obstet Gynecol* 1979; 133:762.

Krebs HB, Petres RE, Dunn LJ, et al: Intrapartum fetal heart rate monitoring: II. Multifactorial analysis of intrapartum fetal heart rate tracings. *Am J Obstet Gynecol* 1979; 133:773.

Krebs HB, et al: Intrapartum fetal heart rate monitoring: IV. Observations on elective and nonelective fetal heart rate monitoring. *Am J Obstet Gynecol* 1980; 138:213.

Krebs HB, Petres RE, Dunn LJ, et al: Intrapartum fetal heart rate monitoring: VI. Prognostic significance of accelerations. *Am J Obstet Gynecol* 1982; 142:297.

Krebs HB, Petres RE, Dunn LJ: Intrapartum fetal heart rate monitoring: VII. Atypical variable decelerations. *Am J Obstet Gynecol* 1983; 145:297.

Lubli F: Impact of intrapartum monitoring on perinatal mortality and morbidity. *Contra Gynecol* 1969; 104:1190.

Lubli FW, Hon EH, Khazin AF, et al: Observations on heart rate and pH in the human fetus during labor. *Am J Obstet Gynecol* 1979; 133:779.

Ledger WJ: Complications associated with invasive monitoring. *Semin Perinatol* 1978; 2:187–194.

Lee CY, Di Loreto RC, O'Lane JM: A study of fetal heart rate acceleration patterns. *Obstet Gynecol* 1975; 45:142.

Leveno KJ, Quirk JG, Cunningham FG, et al: Prolonged pregnancy: I. Observations concerning the causes of fetal distress. *Am J Obstet Gynecol* 1984; 150:465.

Low JA, Cox MJ, Karchmar EJ, et al: The prediction of intrapartum fetal metabolic acidosis by fetal heart rate monitoring. *Am J Obstet Gynecol* 1981; 139:299.

Low JA, Cox MJ, Karchmar EJ, et al: The prediction of intrapartum fetal metabolic acidosis by fetal heart-rate monitoring. *Am J Obstet Gynecol* 1981; 139:299.

Lumley J, McKinnon L, Wood C: Lack of agreement of normal values for fetal scalp blood. *Br J Obstet Gynaecol* 1971; 78:13–21.

MacDonald D, Grant A, Sheridan-Pereira M, et al: The Dublin randomized controlled trial of intrapartum fetal heart rate monitoring. *Am J Obstet Gynecol* 1985; 152:524–539.

Martin CB Jr: Behavioral states in the human fetus. *J Reprod Med* 1981; 26:425–432.

Martin CB: Physiology and clinical use of fetal heart rate variability. *Clin Perinatol* 1982; 9:339.

Martin CB Jr: Regulation of the fetal heart rate and genesis of FHR patterns. *Semin Perinatol* 1978; 2:131–146.

Martin CB, de Haan J, van der Wildt B, et al: Mechanisms of late decelerations in the fetal heart rate: A study with autonomic blocking agents in fetal lambs. *Eur J Obstet Gynaecol Reprod Biol* 1979; 9:361.

Mendez-Bauer C, Poseiro JJ, Arellano-Hernandez G, et al: Effects of atropine on the heart rate of the human fetus during labour. *Am J Obstet Gynecol* 1963; 85:1033.

Mendez-Bauer C, et al: Early deceleration of the fetal heart rate from occlusion of the umbilical cord. *J Perinatal Med* 1978; 6:69.

Miller FC, Sacks DA, Yeh SY, et al: Significance of meconium during labor. *Am J Obstet Gynecol* 1975; 122:573.

Miyazaki FS, Nevarez F: Saline amnioinfusion for relief of repetitive variable decelerations: A prospective randomized study. *Am J Obstet Gynecol* 1985; 153:301–306.

Mueller-Heubach E, et al: Effects of electronic fetal heart rate monitoring on perinatal outcome and obstetric practices. *Am J Obstet Gynecol* 1980; 137:758.

Myers RE, Mueller-Heubach E, Adamsons K: Predictability of the state of fetal oxygenation from a quantitative analysis of the components of late deceleration. *Am J Obstet Gynecol* 1973; 115:1083.

Myers RE: Two patterns of perinatal brain damage and their conditions of occurrence. *Am J Obstet Gynecol* 1972; 112:245.

Mavot D, Mor-Yosef S, Granat M, et al: Antepartum fetal heart rate pattern associated with congenital malformations. *Obstet Gynecol* 1984; 63:414–417.

Nelson KB, Ellenberg JH: Antecedents of cerebral palsy: Multivariate analysis of risk. *N Engl J Med* 1986; 315:81–86.

Painter MJ, Depp R, O'Donoghue PD: Fetal heart rate patterns and development in the first year of life. *Am J Obstet Gynecol* 1979; 132:271–277.

Painter MJ, Scott M, Deep R: Neurological and developmental follow-up of children at 6 to 9 years relative to intrapartum fetal heart rate patterns, in *Fifth Annual Clinical, Scientific, and Business Meetings.* Las Vegas, The Society of Perinatal Obstetricians, Feb 24, 1985.

Parer JT: Effects of atropine on heart rate and oxygen consumption of the hypoxic fetus. *Gynecol Invest* 1977; 8:50.

Parer JT: FHR Monitoring: Answering the critics. *Contemp Obstet Gynecol* 1981; 17:163–174.

Parer JT: The current role of intrapartum fetal scalp sampling. *Clin Obstet Gynecol* 1980; 23:565.

Parer JT, Krueger TR, Harris JL: Fetal oxygen consumption and mechanisms of heart rate response during artificially produced late decelerations of fetal heart rate in sheep. *Am J Obstet Gynecol* 1980; 136:478–482.

Parer JT: The effect of atropine on heart rate and oxygen consumption of the hypoxic fetus. *Am J Obstet Gynecol* 1984; 148:1118–1122.

Patrick J, Carmichael L, Chess L, et al: The distribution of accelerations of the human fetal heart rate at 38 to 40 weeks' gestational age. *Am J Obstet Gynecol* 1985; 151:283–287.

Patrick J, Carmichael L, Chess L, et al: Accelerations of the human fetal heart rate at 38 to 40 weeks' gestational age. *Am J Obstet Gynecol* 1984; 148:35–45.

Paul R, Hon E: Clinical fetal monitoring: V. Effect on perinatal outcome. *Am J Obstet Gynecol* 1974; 118:529–533.

Paul RH, Suidan AK, Yeh S, et al: Clinical fetal monitoring: VII. The evaluation and significance of intrapartum baseline FHR variability. *Am J Obstet Gynecol* 1975; 123:206.

Perkins RP: Sudden fetal death in labor: The significance of antecedent monitoring characteristics and clinical circumstances. *J Reprod Med* 1980; 25:309.

Petrie RH, Yeh S, Murata Y, et al: The effects of drugs on fetal heart rate variability. *Am J Obstet Gynecol* 1978; 130:294.

Pinkerton J: Kergaradec, friend of Laennec and pioneer of fetal auscultation. *Proc R Soc Med* 1969; 62:477–483.

Reece EA, Chervenak FA, Romero R: Magnesium sulfate in the management of acute intrapartum distress. *Am J Obstet Gynecol* 1984; 148:104.

Renou P, Chang A, Anderson I, et al: Controlled trial of fetal intensive care. *Am J Obstet Gynecol* 1976; 126:470–476.

Renou P, Newman W, Wood C: Autonomic control of fetal heart rate. *Am J Obstet Gynecol* 1969; 195:949.

Ron M, Adoni A, Hochner D, et al: The significance of baseline tachycardia in the postterm fetus. *Int J Gynaecol Obstet* 1980; 28:76.

Roversi GD, Cannussio V, Spennacchio M: Recognition and significance of maternogenic fetal acidosis during intensive monitoring of labor. *J Perinatal Med* 1975; 3:53–63.

Sadovsky E, Rabinowitz R, Freeman A, et al: The relationships between fetal heart rate accelerations, fetal movements, and uterine contractions. *Am J Obstet Gynecol* 1984; 149:187–189.

Saling E: Fetal scalp blood analysis. *J Perinatal Med* 1981; 9:157.

Schifferli PY, Caldeyro-Barcia R: Effects of atropine and beta-autonomic drugs on the heart rate of the human fetus, in Boreus L (ed): *Fetal Pharmacology.* New York, Raven, 1973.

Schifrin BS, Shields JR: Perinatal antecedents of cerebral palsy. *Obstet Gynecol* 1988; 71:899–905.

Schifrin BS, Weissman H, Wiley J: Electronic fetal monitoring and obstetrical malpractice, in *Proceedings of Obstetrical Malpractice:* vol 13: *Law, Medicine, and Health Care.* New York, Academy Press, 1984, pp 100–105.

Schifrin BS: Fetal heart rate patterns following epidural anesthesia and oxytocin infusion during labor. *Br J Obstet Gynaecol* 1972; 79:332.

Schifrin BS, Dame L: Fetal heart rate patterns, prediction of Apgar score. *JAMA* 1972; 219:1322–1325.

Shenker L: Fetal cardiac arrhythmias. *Obstet Gynecol Surv* 1979; 34:561–572.

Siassi B, Blanco C, Martin CB: Baroreceptor and chemoreceptor responses to umbilical cord occlusion in fetal lambs. *Biol Neonate* 1979; 35:66–73.

Terao T, Kawashima Y, Noto H, et al: Neurological control of fetal heart rate in 20 cases of anencephalic fetuses. *Am J Obstet Gynecol* 1984; 149:201–208.

Tejani N, Mann L, Bhakthavathsalan A, et al: Correlation of fetal heart rate—uterine contraction patterns with fetal scalp blood pH. *Obstet Gynecol* 1975; 46:392.

Tejani N, Mann L, Bhakthavathsalan A, et al: Prolonged fetal bradycardia with recovery: Its significance and outcome. *Am J Obstet Gynecol* 1975; 122:975.

Tejani N, Schulman H, Fleischer A, et al: The value of quantitative analysis of fetal heart rate tracings. *Perinatol-Neonatol* 1983; 7:55.

Turbeville DF, McCaffree MA: Fetal scalp electrode complications: Cerebrospinal fluid leak. *Obstet Gynecol* 1979; 54:469–470.

Tushuizen PBT, Sloot JEGM, Ubachs JMH: Fetal heart rate monitoring of the dying fetus. *Am J Obstet Gynecol* 1974; 120:922.

van der Moer PE, Gerretsen G, Visser GHA: Fixed fetal heart rate pattern after intrauterine accidental decerebration. *Obstet Gynecol* 1985; 65:125.

Vintzileos AM, Campbell WA, Dreiss RJ, et al: Intrapartum fetal heart rate monitoring of the extremely premature fetus. *Am J Obstet Gynecol* 1985; 151:744.

Visser GHA, Goodman JDS, Levine DH, et al: Diurnal and other cyclic variations in human fetal heart rate near term. *Am J Obstet Gynecol* 1982; 142:535.

Visser GHA, Zeelenberg HJ, De Vries JIP, et al: External physical stimulation of the human fetus during episodes of low heart rate variation. *Am J Obstet Gynecol* 1983; 145:579–584.

Walker NF: Reliability of the signs of fetal distress. *S Afr Med J* 1975; 49:1732.

Westgren M, Ingemarsson E, Ingermarsson I, et al: Intrapartum electronic fetal monitoring in low-risk pregnancies. *Obstet Gynecol* 1980; 56:301.

Wolf S: Central autonomic influences on cardiac rate and rhythm. *Mod Concepts Cardiovasc Dis* 1969; 38:29–34.

Wolfson RN, Sorokin Y, Rosen MG: Autonomic control of fetal cardiac activity, in Elkayam U, Gleicher N (eds): *Cardiac Problems in Pregnancy: Diagnosis and Management of Maternal and Fetal Disease*. New York, Alan R Liss, p 365.

Wood C: Fetal scalp sampling: Its place in management. *Semin Perinatol* 1979; 2:169.

Wood C, Ferguson R, Leeton J, et al: Fetal heart rate in relation to fetal scalp blood measurements in the assessment of fetal hypoxia. *Am J Obstet Gynecol* 1967; 98:62.

Wood C, et al: A controlled trial of fetal heart rate monitoring in a low risk obstetric population. *Am J Obstet Gynecol* 1981; 141:527.

Yeh SY, Zanini B, Petrie RH, et al: Intrapartum fetal cardiac arrest: A preliminary observation. *Obstet Gynecol* 1977; 50:571.

Young BK, Katz M, Klein SA, et al: Fetal blood and tissue pH with moderate bradycardia. *Am J Obstet Gynecol* 1979; 135:45.

Young BK, Katz M, Klein SA: The relationship of heart rate patterns and tissue pH in the human fetus. *Am J Obstet Gynecol* 1979; 134:685.

Young BK, Katz M, Wilson SJ: Sinusoidal fetal heart rate: I. Clinical significance. *Am J Obstet Gynecol* 1980; 136:587–593.

Zalar RW, Quilligan EJ: The influence of fetal scalp sampling on the cesarean section rate for fetal distress. *Am J Obstet Gynecol* 1979; 135:239.

Zanini B, Paul RH, Huey JR: Intrapartum fetal heart rate: Correlation with scalp pH in the preterm fetus. *Am J Obstet Gynecol* 1980; 136:43–47.

Index

in stillbirth, 134
   unexplained, 72
Tachysystole, 78, 80
  in abruptio placentae, 150
  after oxytocin, 166
  in stillbirth, 158
Terbutyline, 17
Tetany, 84
Tocolytics: beta-mimetic, 82
Tranquilizers, 17
Transducers: external, 9
Transfusion: fetal-maternal, 122
Transverse lie, 30
Trendelenburg position, 88, 106

U

Ultrasound, 24
Umbilical
  blood flow impairment in asphyxia, 9
  cord
    compression, 92
    knot causing stillbirth, 146
    nuchal, with maternal fever, 166
    nuchal, around neck, 104
    presentation, 30
Undershooting, 26, 74

Uterus
  activity
    after epidural block, 42
    after paracervical block, 38, 52
    in supine and lateral positions, 36
  anomaly with preterm labor, 148
  blood flow impairment in asphyxia, 9
  hypertonus, 66, 78, 80
    in epidural anesthesia, 90
    paracervical block bradycardia and, 52
  with tetany, 84

V

"Vagal" patterns, 104, 112
Vaginal bleeding: in abruptio placentae, 150

X

Xylocaine, 52